Smoking and Common Sense

Smoking and Common Sense

One Doctor's View

Dr Tage Voss

Edited by
Paul Redfern

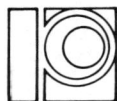

PETER OWEN • *London*

PETER OWEN PUBLISHERS
73 Kenway Road London SW5 0RE

First published in Great Britain 1992
© Tage Voss 1990
Translated from the Danish by Johan Sonne Mortensen
English edition revised and edited by Paul Redfern
English edition © Paul Redfern 1992

A catalogue record for this book is
available from the British Library

ISBN 0 7206 0856 2

Printed in Great Britain by Billings of Worcester

Contents

Tables

Figures

It has been proven beyond any shadow of doubt that smoking is a preferred cause of statistics.

Anonymous

Foreword

In writing this book I have been driven by common sense, tempered with scepticism. My underlying question has been: can it really be true that . . . ?

When people argue about smoking they quote so-called 'scientific facts'. But, strictly speaking, these are opinions based on data which most of us never see and cannot check, and which, therefore, should not be used as gospel truth. The media then repeat these statements uncritically. There is so much debate on the subject that practically anything can be said with little fear of contradiction – as long as it follows the establishment line.

As a physician, my medical education was a practical one, later supplemented by extensive experience of social medicine. But in some of the more esoteric areas of science that have been brought into the tobacco debate I am like a lost child: the subtleties of ventilation technology; building materials pollution; toxicology; forensic analyses of air, blood, and urine; the mathematics of epidemiology; the mysteries of advanced statistics: all these are Greek to me. I am able to work my way through most of them, and that is all.

Such limited understanding is not enough to enable me to be fair to both sides of the debate. But it happens that there is so little agreement between specialists, and so many contradictory findings being published, that very few statements are allowed to stand undisputed for long. The debate is fuelled with a plethora of arguments and counter-arguments, test results and conflicting data. As you follow it, you can always find some specialist to confirm your own scepticism about improbable and arrogant statements.

A great deal is quite simple, however, and therefore not beyond common sense.

When the Danish Health Department's Tobacco Risk Council announces that in the next twelve months 10,000 Danes will die as a result of tobacco smoking, you can take a look at the statistics, and see that the total number of deaths in Denmark is 55,000 per year.

Is it really possible that one out of five Danes will smoke himself to death – considering that one out of two Danes is a non-smoker?

And supposing all these 10,000 had been non-smokers, and therefore could not have died from tobacco smoking, would none of them have died, and would the death rate drop to 45,000 per year? Can this really be true? (And would it be desirable?)

I also wonder how they can claim that so many die as a result of tobacco smoking, when after forty-five years of general practice I have not had a single patient die from this cause; indeed, I have not even heard of any – until recently.

During my work on this book (and long before that) notes, photocopies, extracts, and thick scientific volumes have been piled high on my old desk and have spread over all my window-sills and floor. I mention all this literature only to show how diligent I have been – and to show that I have not made it all up myself.

Some of these articles and books are listed at the end of this volume. I doubt if one in a hundred readers will make any use of them, but if anyone does want to, the sources are there. There are an awful lot of them, and it is impossible for any one person to read them all. I quote only a few of the many sources I have read – but each of these leads one on *ad lib* – sometimes *ad nauseam*: as is the way with scientists, fifty pages of text are often followed by as many pages of references.

Although there is an immense amount of literature, reliable researchers are always coming to the conclusion that we know too little to be able to give final, categorical statements about the effects of smoking, and of passive smoking. Estimates, suppositions and unproven theories dominate the debate – they are the result of belief rather than science. The propaganda against tobacco is characterized by a religious zeal more than by sober objectivity.

So, although it is said to be pointless discussing belief with believers – 'never discuss religion or politics' – you may well be provoked into it when the belief is so aggressively proselytized from such a dubious basis. Hence this book.

Tage Voss

Note: Many of the figures in this book are reprinted, with thanks, from published papers and such sources are acknowledged. Others, however, are simply illustrative of general relationships and are in the spirit of scribbles on a blackboard or the back of an envelope to clarify a point. They are used in this way by Dr Voss in his lectures. (*Ed.*)

Introduction
A Personal Note

The first time I took part in the tobacco debate was in 1958 when the Danish newspaper *Politiken* published my article 'Cancer and Tobacco – Lies and Logic'. I had become annoyed with unfounded (as I saw it) and aggressive interference in people's personal habits: not least by the distorted reasons for this interference, and the lack of logic. We are, apparently, not a single step further forward today.

Over the next thirty years this subject became a favourite topic for discussion in the media. The arguments have not improved, and the 'facts' are as over-interpreted as ever. Now the question of passive smoking has been introduced and the anti-smokers have formed an international lobby which has great influence on authorities and on legislation, so that smokers are not only made to feel unwanted, but in some places downright criminal. The basis of the lobby is still a distortion of the facts, with an oblique shift in the priorities given to health problems, and a very aggressive stance.

My tolerance . . .

I hope I am a tolerant person, but when I recall how the Nazis perverted public opinion and intimidated dissidents, I feel that I must react sharply against attempts to influence legislation and attitudes through pressure and threats. That I am a smoker myself (though not of the discredited cigarette) has, of course, added weight to my instinct to fight this limitation of people's freedom to choose their own lifestyle.

I find it a little ridiculous that any reasonable person should have to waste time considering the problem of tobacco, a trivial matter in a world where we are threatened with annihilation from global catastrophes. There should be far more important things in the world to worry about than tobacco. Nobody recognizes this more clearly than I do. I interpret the tobacco debate as a symptom of authoritarianism, and find it as essential to react against it as against any kind of manipulation, threat to human integrity, or abrogation of individual freedom.

I have smoked for more than fifty years and I have never given the matter a thought – other than as a pleasant experience, adding a little spice to my life. It has never been a problem for me, and I have no reason to believe that my smoking has been a problem for anybody else. When in middle age I used to visit my elderly parents, our meetings would always end with my father's invitation: 'Well, son, let's have a good cigar.' We did, and were able to handle all the problems of the world while the blue smoke circled towards the ceiling.

My mother never smoked, but she didn't mind other people doing so, possibly because in their early years my family was poor, and never became particularly well off. A cigar was a symbol of luxury, an excuse for a little extravagance, and my mother was pleased when my father could enjoy this small intimation of wealth.

In a home movie I have kept, you can see her tenderly fanning the smoke from my father's newly lit cigar towards her, so that she could sniff it and share the pleasure with him (they were then around seventy years of age). I often recall this gesture, which I have seen thousands of times during my life, and in the ongoing debate it has made me suspect that the position of passive smokers is conditioned by attitude more than by objective nuisance.

My doubts . . .

The tobacco debate is relatively new. It has arisen suddenly, to the great astonishment of an old smoker who has gone unmolested through life until recently. I have never, I believe, considered smoking healthy – just pleasant. It adds to the quality of life, and it helps you through the bad times. That it should be as unhealthy as anti-smokers now fiercely maintain does not seem plausible to me.

As a physician I have dabbled in scientific problems enough to know that in statistical analysis conclusions should not be drawn from small samples. However, I must tell you my reasons for my own relaxed attitude to the anti-smoking hysteria.

I cannot help but doubt the validity of claims that smoking tobacco leads to cancer, heart disease, and early death; that tobacco smoke is damaging, indeed dangerous. Throughout my years as a physician I have treated thousands of patients, but I never had the impression that their complaints derived *specifically* from smoking, nor that they could be treated successfully with a ban on smoking. It is quite another matter that certain diseases of the air passages in the nose, throat, and chest are unlikely to benefit from tobacco smoke, and advice can be given to that effect.

Too many smokers reach the ages predicted by life expectancy charts in fine condition to convince me that smoking is so terribly dangerous, or even a threat to health; many round-shouldered persistent wheezers have never smoked tobacco. To be blunt, the causal connection is unclear.

My family . . .

My entire family had lifelong exposure to tobacco smoke, smoked directly or inhaled in smoke-filled drawing rooms and bars. None of them had heart trouble and none got lung cancer. They all lived to a great age and, to my knowledge, never missed work because of illness. My father's family were mostly artisans, my aunts were married to artisans; all of them lived in the city of Copenhagen. My grandfather came from Holstein, spoke broken Danish, and was never seen without a cigar sticking out of his short beard. He died at the age of eighty-six with a big Brazil in his mouth. On Sundays and at parties, I had enough uncles to

man three card tables in the study, and there were even more
who did not participate, but everyone smoked cigars, all the
time. All of them reached an advanced age, appeared to have
excellent lungs, and died of old age.

Grandmother did not smoke, but most of my aunts did. The
younger ones smoked cigarettes (then mostly Egyptians), the
older ones cheroots, Aunt Hanne even big cigars. During these
gatherings the rooms were thick with tobacco smoke, and by late
evening we children had to take a bearing on the doors from
memory, to get to them through the deepening fog. Nobody
complained; that was simply the way it was. We had our childhood diseases, which we managed to survive, and we thrived –
indeed, more than that after the discovery of vitamins. Cousin
Inger died from tuberculosis, but no member of my family ever
got lung cancer or cardiovascular disease.

I have a photograph of my father at the age of eighty-five
smoking a Havana Corona: 28,000 cigars later he died at ninety-
three, with lungs like a horse and no heart complaints.

The only 'sickly' person was Aunt Amanda, the sister of an
uncle by marriage, a neurotic woman who suffered alternately
from headaches, backaches, cystitis, palpitation, sleeplessness,
and a lot more, by way of which she made strong appeals for
compassion from those around her. She was divorced, lived
alone, and – *mirabile dictu* – she did not smoke. But she was never
so ill that she missed out on a family reunion – and she never
complained about any nuisance from tobacco smoke.

My mother's relatives were civil servants, book-keepers,
teachers, and one journalist. They also smoked cigars like my
maternal grandfather, but not so intensely – my aunts hardly at
all. Their lifespan was between seventy and eighty years, where-
as my father's family averaged between eighty and ninety. It has
never occurred to me before that this could be connected to the
difference in smoking habits. It might. But inherited character-
istics provide a more likely explanation.

My scepticism . . .

Nowadays, it is alleged that smoking is dangerous to our health. I do not dismiss the possibility that this may be true for some people, but such general statements can hardly be regarded as valid without reservations. 'Tobacco smoking leads to lung cancer' has to be modified – since it almost never does[1] – to 'Tobacco smoking may contribute to some cases of lung cancer' – which is too long and indefinite a sentence for cigarette packets, and too vague as a slogan.[2]

My scepticism towards this kind of unqualified allegation is not based entirely on my own observations. Common sense tells me that physiological truth cannot be *that* simple. And a closer examination of the scientific material, on which the crude assertions of the campaign against tobacco are supposedly based, shows how facts get distorted, how biased and dubious test results are interpreted, and how cheerfully individual findings are generalized.

The success of the campaign is partly due to the fact that the documentation is difficult to understand and inaccessible to most of those at whom it is directed: the general public, readers, viewers, the man in the street; everybody who either smokes or doesn't smoke because they themselves have chosen this lifestyle – which they are obviously not allowed to do any longer, because 'we' insist that they should do something else.

Why. . .?

My objectivity . . .

Almost all scientific literature about smoking and passive smoking is either published in English, or in other languages with

1. Only around one-tenth of smokers contract lung cancer – whatever its cause. (*Ed.*)

2. The UK voluntary agreement between cigarette manufacturers and the Government requires one of six warnings to be printed on packets. They include: '*Smoking can cause fatal diseases*'; '*Smoking can cause lung cancer, bronchitis and other chest diseases*'; and '*More than 30,000 people die each year in the UK from lung cancer*'. (*Ed.*)

English summaries. So anyone who is not English is at the mercy
of all sorts of interpretations and propaganda on the subject.
Even English-speakers are unlikely to have access to the literature itself – or the energy to pursue it. This is the reason why the
anti-smokers always seem to have an easy job getting their
broadsides published. Faced with the authority of the printed
word and the power of repetition, public opinion can offer
nothing in return except a general scepticism and common sense.
Is this enough to counter some of the harsher attacks on tobacco and the propaganda against the poor smokers' peaceful
pleasure?

Scepticism alone is not enough. To strengthen sceptics' doubts
about the 'facts' behind this authoritarian protectiveness, I offer
you an objective review of the problems. And this English
language version is, I discover, as necessary as the Danish
original: being able to read the US Surgeon General's report in
English doesn't mean that anyone actually does – not even the
journalists who pick up the press releases.

So this book contains my own attempt to balance the facts; it
gives an account of the difficulties and doubts connected with
measurements and calculations in this field, and explains why it
is so difficult to produce reliable, unambiguous statements about
the dangers and risks related to both smoking and passive
smoking.

My own astonishment at the number of allegations made
about the lethal effects of tobacco has led me to consider as many
of these as possible. As a physician I have had no difficulty
gaining access to most of those scientific works that anti-smokers
refer to as proof of their allegations. Managing to read all of them
has been more tiresome, since they number many hundreds and
more are being published all the time.

There are more than one thousand scientific publications or
papers about passive smoking alone. So thank God for the
summaries, which have made it possible to avoid the detailed
reading of uninteresting material, and to weed out the irrelevant
and the repetitious. Each time a horrifying assertion about the
danger of tobacco is published in the professional or daily press
('A Dutch researcher has demonstrated that children of smoking

parents have a death rate four times higher than . . .') it has been interesting to search out the Dutch researcher's paper and try to assess its validity. It often turns out that colleagues have done this already, and have expressed their qualified doubts about quality, methodology, and interpretation. But the assertions are still repeated as though they were true. Where doubts have not been cast, we, alone, must generate them about the allegations.

With a surprising frequency, the original publication does not even contain the 'quotation'. We learn how necessary it is to approach such 'quotations' with reservation, and how tendentiously – and irresponsibly – quotations are chosen for propaganda purposes.

1

The Crusade against Tobacco

In recent years, the campaign against tobacco has intensified to the point that it has become venomous. It is in the nature of a crusade, because it is dogmatic and one-sided rather than scientific in character. Drastic measures are implemented, and the smoker is treated more and more aggressively – with hatred even. And, with a strange lack of resistance, the measures are translated into legislation and prohibition, with increasing severity in many areas.

The US Surgeon General

One fanatical anti-smoker was, for instance, the recently retired US Surgeon General, Dr Everett Koop. In the name of health, he launched his salvos against tobacco smoking in the annual reports of the US Health Administration. These reports are not scientific publications, but recommendations of a policy advocated by the health service. Anything which can be said in support of this policy is stated; anything against it is overlooked. Unfortunately, the US Surgeon General's reports are viewed as authoritative, and are uncritically reported in all countries as if they are creeds – perhaps totems of the New Age. Dr Koop left his position late in 1989, and perhaps we may now look forward to future reports from a physician with a more balanced attitude, perhaps even a happy tobacco smoker himself.

WHO

The World Health Organization (WHO) also publishes recommendations which are supposed to inspire respectful governments to take action against tobacco smoking. Even the EC pursues a militant policy, demanding prohibition, restrictions, and propaganda offensives against tobacco. Everything is done to protect European citizens and to live up to the programme of 'Health for All by the Year 2000'.

Unfortunately, this is precisely the way to exacerbate the conflict with smokers, who may not feel that their health is being damaged, who are not convinced that these vehement attacks on their peaceful vice are based on objectivity, and who feel their private life being invaded and victimized by still more aggressive interference.

Most of them have difficulty making sense of WHO's considerable efforts to make people who have chosen to smoke tobacco because they like it, choose again – to quit smoking. WHO's campaign is directed at industrialized countries with high standards of living and an average life expectancy of more than seventy years – at the expense of their efforts for poorer populations with an average life expectancy of less than forty years because of lack of food, poor drinking water, miserable housing conditions, diarrhoea, malaria, tuberculosis, AIDS, bilharzia, and so on.

One cannot help thinking that their efforts should be devoted to giving one third of the world's population a genuine choice between hunger or satiety, between death by untreated disease or life following treatment.

If we're talking about 'Health for All . . .', tobacco smoking in the developed world seems a minor problem.

EC

The authorities seem to have taken sides, no matter what their basis is for doing so. It did not come from science. The EC Commission want a directive (moved before the Council on

7 April 1989) harmonizing tobacco advertising, 'out of consideration for the health of all citizens, especially the young'. They
refer to the European Council's action programme for fighting
cancer, and want to contribute to the improvement of European
citizens' health status and quality of life, by reducing the number
of cancer cases. They therefore put a high priority on limiting the
consumption of tobacco.

This is to be implemented by special warnings printed on all
tobacco advertisements in the press, and on posters as well as
wrappings and packings. The list of warnings comprises 12
phrases, for instance: 'Smoking leads to cancer', 'Smoking leads
to cardiovascular diseases', 'Smokers die early', 'Smoking kills
you', 'Smoking leads to deadly diseases' – all terrible threats and
categorical statements.

The concern does not stop here. The matter has been sent to
the Committee for Environment, Health and Consumer Protec-
tion, who moved an amendment to the European Parliament on
7 February 1990 extending the directive to films and other media
'and in connection with sponsored events'. The proposal forbids
all kinds of tobacco advertising, as Portugal and Italy have
already done. A ban on every kind of indirect advertising is also
to be introduced. 'Member states having not yet introduced
prohibition, should forbid every kind of advertisement for tobacco in every kind of publication.' The argument is based on
concern for the general public's health.

There is yet another proposition – to amend the amendment –
from the Committee for Youth, Culture, Education, Media and
Sports, who demand ever more stringent prohibitions – dictating
the size and placing of the warnings on tobacco packaging, and
organizing information campaigns in schools, in the armed
forces, and on television about the dangers of tobacco smoking.
The lower you get in subcommittees, the more unconditional
and polemical are the statements, and the less responsible in
terms of the use of factual evidence.

This obsessive concern for health appears in a different per-
spective when one remembers that in Denmark, for instance,
the impact of occupational injuries and occasional poisoning
accidents with paint, household articles, and solvents resulted

eventually in an injunction about labelling such articles with danger categories and warnings about the possibility of poisoning. The measure was later suspended after objections from the EC, who considered that it hindered free competition and the unimpeded distribution of goods inside the inner market. Considerations of health do not weigh equally from case to case!

Danish Medical Ethics Council

There are many examples of intimidation and hate campaigns against those who stand up in public in defence of a little common sense and a more balanced view on tobacco. In 1988 an action was brought against me at the Danish Medical Ethics Council by one of the militant anti-smoker associations as part of their campaign against tobacco smoking. Their complaint was that I, as a doctor, had acted unethically by making public my doubts about the danger of passive smoking, and that I had not (as doctors are supposed to do) taken the trouble to keep up-to-date with the latest research on the subject – which would, it went without saying, demonstrate this danger.

This compelled the Medical Ethics Council to go through the scientific literature to see if there was any support for the allegation that passive smoking is dangerous. Unlike the media, doctors in general do not give tobacco problems a high priority. Many of them smoke themselves and are happy about it, and do not find the supposed dangers to health convincing in relation to so many other threats to health in modern life.[1]

I imagine that my good colleagues in the Medical Ethics Council searched with little enthusiasm through some of the more accessible scientific material on this subject, which as I have already said now comprises more than one thousand papers from all over the world (not all of them equally serious). Having done this the Council reached the same conclusion as I had, and confirmed the truth of my claim that up until then no scientific

1. In the UK most doctors claim not to smoke when questioned in surveys. (*Ed.*)

proof had been produced that passive smoking threatened any-body's health.

This made little or no impression upon those who issued the accusations and made the allegations about the damaging effects of passive smoking. They did not go so far as to bring an action against the Council for unethical behaviour in agreeing with me but, impervious to the ruling, the 'damaging' effects of passive smoking are still a mainstay of their propaganda. That the Medical Ethics Council acquitted me of the accusation changed nothing. My unaltered sceptical attitude to the anti-smoking arguments has even resulted in further hateful public attacks. The chairman of one of the most militant anti-smoking associa-tions, a medical colleague at that, stated with the typical subtlety of the gutter press: 'Smoke yourself to death, Tage Voss. You are a disgrace to the medical profession.' And a journalist who has made tobacco his favourite subject writes that I ought to be thrown out of the medical association!

The means my adversaries choose are not characterized by delicacy, and objective facts still do not get through to the heart of the debate.

Lies and damned lies

The question remains: why do we experience such militant persecution of smokers now – after 300 years of smoking in Europe? Is it to divert public attention away from real threats – or just typical media scare-mongering? Tobacco has been a perennial target for silly season stories, even more so than the Loch Ness monster. The number of column inches devoted to anti-smoking propaganda has been considerable compared with that given to crucial problems concerning ecology or government matters, not to mention potential social, occupational, and en-vironmental menaces.

Is there any real danger in smoking at all, and, if so, can its scope be assessed? Most of the arguments against it are dog-matic, and can be questioned only by running the risk of being considered unreliable or even criminal. But flimsy arguments are no worse for constant repetition, gaining authority each time they are quoted – especially by a willing press.

Each year, in Denmark, 25,000 smokers die. Has this kind of figure any meaning at all? Every year, 30,000 *non*-smokers and 20,000 drivers die. But, of the whole population, four-fifths die at a great age. Most drivers do not die because they are drivers, nor do non-smokers die because they are non-smokers. And of the smokers 23,000 die each year without contracting lung cancer.

We learned from Dr Goebbels that you do not necessarily have to falsify figures to be able to use them successfully in your propaganda. Army reports about formidable numbers of destroyed enemy tanks on the Eastern Front gave an encouraging impression of German luck and superiority in the war – as long as the number of lost German tanks was not mentioned.

The technique is still in use today. In a professional journal there is a calculation by Dr Hiroshi Nakajima, who demonstrates that every 13 seconds somewhere in this world a smoker dies. This observation has been discussed in the world press and is put forward as a new argument in the debate by the WHO (to which Dr Nakajima was appointed Secretary-General in the late 1980s). How, then, can anybody justify continuing to smoke? Surely, at the very least, life insurance premiums should be raised for smokers?

Let us mobilize reason, add a little scepticism, mix in O-level maths, and look it up in WHO's *Health Statistics 1988*. We find that the total annual death rate of the world population of 5,112,298,000 is 10.4 per 1000. We can then easily work out that 1.7 people die every second.

But according to Dr Nakajima a smoker dies every 13 seconds. It now looks as though smokers are less at risk than the population at large. So should not more people start smoking for the sake of world health?

However, the possibility of causal connection has not been taken into account. Tobacco smokers die – but how many die of tobacco smoking? Smoking may have as little to do with survival as it may have to do with dying. Some smokers may even die like other people – from old age, or in a traffic accident.

Recently there was a report from Italy about the children of smoking parents apparently snoring more than non-smokers' children. The press ran headlines like 'Passive smoking makes children ill' and 'Smokers' children snore the most'. The stories suggested that snoring may be a very serious matter, connected to increased blood pressure, cardiac problems and strokes. The risk of these conditions in children seems, to say the least, a little bit exaggerated. Apart from this, what does the text say? Seven out of ten snoring Italian children had parents who smoked tobacco! But it does not say that nine out of ten snoring Italian children had parents who ate spaghetti. The error is to present coincidence as evidence of causation.

The influence of social conditions

When it is stated as fact that children of smoking parents more often have inflammation of the ear, bronchitis, and head colds, nothing is said about cause and effect. Nothing suggests that the increased sickliness of these children is caused exclusively by their parents' smoking, as we are cunningly led to believe.

Nor is it mentioned that this does not hold good generally, and does not concern all children of smoking parents. If there are, for instance, nine cases of illness per month among children in a group of non-smoking families and ten in an equally large group of smoking families, then it is supposed to be demonstrated that children of smoking parents are more often sick! We need to be told the absolute size of the groups: perhaps there were no sick children at all in nine out of ten smoking families.

Nothing is said about 'confounding factors'[2] that can blur the picture and affect results. It has been clearly demonstrated that smoking in the UK is more frequent among the lower social groups, where there are also lower levels of hygiene, housing standards, nourishment, and child care. It is precisely those illnesses mentioned above that are characteristically more frequent

---

2. 'Confounding factors': a term used by epidemiologists to designate all other physical, sociological, or psychological elements that have been shown to be associated with the risk criteria under study. (*Ed.*)

in low status groups. It seems peculiar that this huge concern for the health of children apparently neglects housing conditions and concentrates exclusively on parents' smoking.

I doubt that the effect of parental cigarette smoking in a single-family house with a nursery and a garden could have the same influence on a child's health as in a two-room flat in a crowded inner city slum. We certainly need a correction for housing conditions as well as social status in any discussion on the influence of tobacco smoking.

We have also failed to take note of other circumstances. There is cross-infection: from sick parents, snuffling children in nursery school, elderly coughing relatives, ill siblings. Hereditary conditions may have an influence on the frequency of such illnesses. Moreover, children are usually away from home between break-fast and teatime. During this period the children can scarcely be influenced by the smoking habits of their parents. We may assume also that few parents smoke at night while they are asleep.

It has been estimated in Denmark that most children now spend only an hour and a half during the day in the company of their parents. If that is indeed the case, surely it is more important to their health where they spend the rest of the day: the amount of exhaust fumes they breathe, and how damaging the indoor air is in those institutions where they spend so much of the day.

Parental smoking is thus an extremely unlikely cause of children's illnesses. Nevertheless it is repeatedly put forward as a weighty charge against smoking. As with parental smoking, so it is with other well-worn arguments in the campaign against tobacco; there is much that is sheer nonsense.

A major health threat?

On 21 December 1989 a press release from a Scandinavian group coordinating the fight against cancer said that it had decided to concentrate all its efforts on stopping people smoking, as 'the main part of the 100,000 annual cases of cancer in the Scandinavian countries is due to smoking'.

Every year 250,000 people die in Scandinavia. The cancer toll is 23 per cent of all deaths.[3] Consequently, in Scandinavia there will be 57,500 cases of death from cancer annually.

The slogan for the campaign gives the number of cancer *cases* as 100,000, while the number of cancer *deaths* is 57,500 at the most. Thus the public is being fooled, without being lied to directly. But cancers that remit spontaneously, are cured by treatment, or are wrongly diagnosed and therefore not cancer at all, are to me on a level with other non-fatal diseases. The number of cancer patients either cured or dying from other causes such as heart failure, traffic accidents, or suicide, will not be registered as cancer deaths, and are not cancer deaths. So a diagnosis of cancer for this latter group becomes irrelevant. Is it reasonable to quote the number of cancer cases in a scare campaign, and then afterwards admit that this figure is really only half as terrifying? Yet this is being done.

Let us look more closely at the figures. So far, nobody has suggested that bone cancer is caused by smoking, nor that cancer of the liver, intestines, breast, skin, prostate, or uterus are caused by smoking. That leaves cancer of the respiratory organs, mainly the lungs. In Scandinavia there are approximately 13,000 lung cancer deaths per year, of which 20 to 25 per cent (3,000), unjustly enough, strike at non-smokers. Autopsies show, though, that 25 per cent of cancers found in lungs are adenocarcinomas, a cancer form seldom originating in the lungs but sometimes spreading to them from other organs.

That leaves 7,500 deaths from primary lung cancer among smokers. Eighty-two per cent of these affect people over sixty years of age, a group in which the general mortality rate increases rapidly. In this group prolonged survival is unlikely to be based on eliminating a single cause of death. Finally, lung cancer is well known to be multi-factorial: it has many different, often interdependent causes, and the main one can be determined only in special cases. It is disingenuous to claim tobacco smoking as the primary cause of lung cancer.

So, the target group of the Scandinavian Fight-Against-Cancer

3. Danish Health Administration, *Cause of Death Statistics 1987.*

campaign is now seen to be reduced to a little over 1,500 smokers under 60 years of age – 0.075 per thousand Scandinavians. All that is left for the campaigners to prove is that these 1,500 will *not* contract lung cancer if they stop smoking. Plus, of course, that they will not die from other causes – especially if they are delicate, socially underprivileged, afflicted with an hereditary illness, drug abusers, diabetics, spastics, epileptics, or psychiatric patients. This will be difficult, if not impossible.

When, therefore, the Management of the Scandinavian Fight-Against-Cancer decided 'to concentrate all efforts in 1990 on the fight against tobacco smoking' by attempting to brainwash 20 million people, it cannot be said to be on the basis of statistics nor, for that matter, on the basis of medical facts. On what basis, then?

As I hope I have shown, the objective basis is indeed weak. The campaigners play on the public's fear, and make cancer the life-threatening bogyman in twice as many cases as the reality; illogically they also imply that there is a causal connection between smoking and the many different types of cancer. But even when 'facts' have been shown to be false, the political demagoguery by the health lobby continues indefatigably – morally and economically supported by public funds, and by . . . well, by what else?

2
Active Smoking and Passive Smoking

The two separate components of the tobacco debate – active smoking and passive smoking – are not always kept apart. The result is much confusion and a good deal of nonsense. Most commonly, research into the effects of active smoking is brought into the debate on the effects of passive smoking. But these effects are from quite different concentrations of the suspect substances as well as, partly, from different substances.

The most honest debaters make clear whether they are talking about active smoking or passive smoking. Many are not so honest, and some are just not aware of any difference.

The question is really very simple. To smoke or not to smoke is the choice an individual makes between immediate pleasure and possible future harmful effects. If smoking is a threat to health, and if this fact is not kept a secret, then it must be up to the individual to choose for himself how to act. This is not very different from choosing between yachting or motor rallying, or between beef and beans. It is a private matter, a personal choice. There is no need for outside interference.

In the propaganda campaign against smoking, the debate has been given a new focus by introducing an element of social responsibility: damage to health by smoking costs society money! Nearly three hundred years ago Ludvig Holberg[1] drew attention to other social aspects of tobacco when he pointed out that tobacco smoking gave a brown taint to white walls and often caused fires. These consequences have been ignored in the current

1. Ludvig Holberg (1684–1754) is regarded as the founder of Danish literature. He wrote comic plays and poems, historical works, and essays – a sort of Danish Molière. (*Ed.*)

debate. On the other hand, statistics are fielded on working days lost, sick pay, and insurance expenses to prove that medicines, hospital beds, and the treatment of those affected by smoking costs money.

Compare the costs . . .

Pragmatic evidence does not show that there is any connection between smoking and lost working days. An analysis by the US National Center of Health Statistics on sick leave between 1983 and 1985 (Bonilla) showed that smokers have no more absences than non-smokers. Nor is there any indication that smokers consult GPs more frequently than non-smokers. In contrast, according to official hospital statistics, 'healthy' sporting activities result in ten million medical treatments annually in Denmark, costing the equivalent of £100 million. If national policies were led by social, economic, and moral considerations, football and athletics would be banned long before tobacco smoking was mentioned. Nobody is considering that, are they?

So, to smoke or not to smoke should remain a private decision beyond the bounds of public debate and the interference of bureaucrats.

Passive smoking has become an issue recently, and it is considerably more difficult to clarify. It concerns the inconveniences inflicted on non-smokers by tobacco smoke – which means that it is a social or cultural question, rather than a health one.

The problem has become more pressing now that most people in the developed world spend more time indoors than ever before – often in large groups in the same areas.

During my lifetime, conditions have changed radically. When I was a schoolboy three quarters of the Danish population lived in the country, and most workers in towns were active in the open air on building sites, in tanneries, as municipal workers, drivers, tramway and railway employees, navvies and welders. Factories and homes alike were heated by stoves so there was a continuous flow of air – in through draughty doors and windows and out up the chimneys. The air was renewed frequently.

The ventilation factor

Today, almost everybody works indoors: to a great extent in modern buildings made with unnatural materials like concrete and glass; centrally heated and ventilated by recycling the air to save energy; with no provision for opening the windows or altering the regulated temperature.

The problem of indoor air is persistently underrated. In recent years international conferences on the quality of indoor air have attracted physiologists, physicians, epidemiologists, physicists, building engineers, chemists, and architects. I have taken part in several of them myself, and cover the subject more fully in Chapter 11.

A key problem is to find methods of defining indoor air, and assessing the influence of different factors on humans. How you react physically to the environment is not the only question. There is also the vaguer quality of well-being. How do you feel, how well do you work under certain conditions? It is difficult to find objective measurements for well-being. Sick leave and working efficiency may be an expression of well-being. But what environmental factors are concerned? Humidity, infrasonic oscillations, carbon monoxide, lighting . . .?

If you ask 'What is the most comfortable temperature?' you will get as many different answers as the number of times you ask the question. People's perceptions of hot and cold vary widely within the few degrees' range that we would all accept as normal.

Only when large numbers of staff become seriously ill from a specific infection, such as Legionnaire's disease or Pontiac fever[2], is an unequivocal cause sought and, hopefully, found: in the former case from bacterial infection of the ventilation shafts. These infections afflict at least 40,000 people annually in the United States.

Aside from these high profile outbreaks, any problems people appear to be having are kept on a personal level by management.

---

2. Originally an infection of more than a hundred people employed at the Health Department in Pontiac, Michigan, USA.

If you get ill it is because you are unhealthy; if you do not thrive it is because you are delicate.

It may not be intentional, but this development looks like an abrogation of responsibility for prosperity and health. If the issue of the quality of air inside public buildings, hospitals, schools, and working places is dominated by attempts to eliminate tobacco smoking, then attention is drawn away from other factors that are the responsibility of public authorities and of companies. Think how expensive and difficult it would be for most organizations to provide better indoor air – and see why focusing on smoking helps them to push into the background the need for proper ventilation.

Pollution in the work place – solvents, dust, heat, noise – often has to be tolerated because local authorities and their inspectors bend the limits laid down by experts. If the noise level in a brewery bottling hall does not exceed that established as tolerable for normal human beings and 80 per cent of the workers get defective hearing, the conclusion may be that the 'tolerable' level is too high and should be lowered. It may be, though, that the brewery workers are abnormal (the Brewery Report)[3]. When excessive numbers of decorators frequently exposed to solvents were found to have brain damage (the Painter Report)[4], a couple of prominent physicians suggested that painters are well known for being more stupid than other people!

It is the same with accidents in the workplace. The blame is put on fatigue, carelessness, or the breaking of safety regulations by the workers themselves. This is called 'blaming the victim'.

And it is the same with outdoor air. In Copenhagen the authorities have given up smog alarms, and have now stopped worrying about the levels of lead in the air round children's playgrounds. They seem to have given up trying to deal with industrial and automobile pollution. Acid rain destroys iron-work; exhaust fumes poison the air and kill trees; industrial effluent makes sculptures crumble and the façades of houses collapse: do these things not damage the mucous membranes of

3 and 4. These are often-quoted, but unpublished reports made by Danish medical students. (*Ed.*)

human lungs? Apparently not enough to activate the authorities.

So, if you contract a lung disease, the blame is on you: you smoke tobacco. Blame the victim. . . .

The significance to poor health of low humidity, static electricity, radiant heat from lights, concrete sweat, bacteria and fungus spores from dirty ventilation ducts, fibres from walls, floors, and ceilings, carbon monoxide from boiler rooms and underground car parks, formaldehyde and styrene from glue, ozone from office machines, and radon seeping through the foundations has now been realized by many. But legislature and their inspectorate ignore these factors. In spite of them, the Sick Building Syndrome is discussed all over the world as essentially a problem of health and welfare. Unfortunately, it will be extremely expensive to do anything to improve most existing buildings. And for new buildings cost is more important than human welfare.

Instead, the focus is on tobacco smoking. As it is the one form of pollution that can be seen and smelt, it is easy to make it the scapegoat – indeed, to feature it as the main factor in many minor complaints. Headache, drowsiness, dry mouth and throat, smarting eyes – the bad indoor air must be caused by tobacco smoke.

If you have cause to criticize your indoor air, the first reaction is to say 'Stop smoking'. Yes, but both smokers and non-smokers complain. Then, of course, the complaints of the non-smokers are due to your smoking. How will companies explain it later when the complaints continue after they abolish smoking and lose a scapegoat? Who knows, perhaps they will miss the tobacco smokers!

To smoke or not to smoke, that is the question. The *US Trade Union* magazine says focusing on smoking will mean a serious setback for efforts to protect the health of the American worker. The risks of occupational disease are currently played down and underestimated, with the ridiculous implication that if workers stop smoking tobacco, occupational diseases will have been virtually eliminated.

But in spite of the political overtones, and ignoring the fact that the connection between passive smoking and ill-health is unproven, the crux of the matter is that non-smokers should not be bothered by tobacco smoke, or – at the very least – that the pleasure of smokers is not paid for by inconveniencing non-smokers. This must be discussed and sorted out, all the more so because the indoor environment is more susceptible to pollution than ever before.

The problem is to balance consideration for smokers with tolerance for non-smokers. This supreme challenge to humanity and the ability to compromise falls, I fear, on stony ground. These are hard times; everybody looks after himself, defends his privileges and demands deference to his wishes. The controversy about tobacco smoking has become a token for the loss of friendliness, generosity, and respect.

Courtesy both ways?

As we have seen, the effects of passive smoking cannot be measured properly. The reaction of the individual is the only thing to go by. Consideration for non-smokers has (as in my family) not exactly been at the forefront of our thoughts. The fact is that until recently they have been totally disregarded. But now the pendulum has swung too far the other way, and the demand for consideration is heavily overplayed. Some people express horror and revulsion towards smokers.

It seems it is not enough simply to ask to be spared the nuisance of another's smoking. The debate has to be given a new factor: health considerations.

If non-smokers become ill from exposure to smoking, the result is a heavy moral burden on smokers, who may even be portrayed as criminals. Suddenly, it is no longer a question of non-smokers in canteens. It is 'the health of the nation', 'fellow citizens getting asthma and cancer' from the smoke, 'it is the children'! Smokers certainly get themselves into weak positions, apparently totally untenable ones. So the field belongs to the anti-smokers.

But the problem remains: it must be proved that passive smoking is a threat to health, insofar as the anti-smokers find it necessary to prove anything before they make statements.

Does Environmental Tobacco Smoke, ETS, mean a documented worsening of already polluted air? There are no clear facts here, in spite of many attempts to estimate the contribution of tobacco smoke to indoor air by measuring how much of each suspected substance is in the air. The anti-smokers have to fall back on unproven statements that have become vaguer and vaguer in recent years. It is even more difficult to produce reliable estimates of the *health* effects of ETS. Indeed, it is so difficult that a review by WHO investigators in November 1988 of published work on passive smoking concluded that there was insufficient evidence to be certain about the health aspects of passive smoking.

Among good and decent people, 'I do not like tobacco smoke' has become 'I cannot tolerate tobacco smoke, it makes me ill.' Everybody with hypochondria or a martyr complex is thus invited to demonstrate his agony and sickness from other people's tobacco smoke. It happens. And it puts pressure on colleagues, trade unions, and management by suggesting 'Stop people smoking – or I quit'.

In conditions of high unemployment, companies are free to decide whether they want to fulfil demands about banning smoking in the work place, or to abandon non-smokers. A walk-out of smokers – or non-smokers – can easily be compensated for from the surplus labour force. Employees are made defenceless against management dictates; the issue becomes a problem for the unions; and may easily go to court to be made legal. This is the reason why chief executives tend to give in to forceful demands, and give up the smokers' right to smoke, to avoid trouble, and even to receive the blessings of the authorities as well as pats on the shoulder from whingeing puritans.

Before it gets this far, however, non-smokers have obtained powerful constraints against smokers, who are now in a situation where they must ask for permission to exist. Considerate smokers have in the past surrendered themselves to the tolerance of non-smokers: they have had to say, 'If it doesn't bother anybody, do you mind if we smoke here?' Suppose this tolerance does not exist . . .?

Smoking is not considered a human right. You may have permission if nobody is against it. Nobody? Under these conditions, one anti-smoker may dictate to 100 smokers, to 200 smokers. And this is being done: in the work place, in buses and trains, in waiting rooms, in post offices, in supermarkets, and in town halls.

Are smokers really supposed to be reduced to smoking in the bog like schoolboys? No, because there's 'No Smoking in the Toilets'. The next person caught short could well be a non-smoker who is nauseated by the smell of tobacco smoke. . . .

So the smoker is outlawed and becomes fair game for hunters – with no off-season. If you break the law, the answer is quite simple: dismissal, a fine, or a police baton on the skull. What a beautiful human quality tolerance is in the hands of authority. . . .

The question of reasonable regard for the well-being of non-smokers weighed against the pleasure of smoking is, however, still under debate, unclarified. It's now complicated by an angry ambience in which the smokers' meek defence can no longer cope with the anti-smokers' spiteful attacks.

But, for the time being, the debate about the responsibility for health-threatening indoor air is pleasantly diverted. . . .

3
The Harmful Effects of Smoking

Smoking tobacco is dangerous, they say. The President of the American Cancer Society, Dr H. Pollard, has declared: 'Without smoking, we would not have lung cancer'. Newspaper headlines claim: 'Tobacco kills'. And the law insists cigarette packs carry the slogan 'Smoking Leads to Lung Cancer'.

It is obvious that these claims are incorrect. Many non-smokers (in Denmark 800 a year) die from lung cancer, so we would still have those, in spite of Dr Pollard. The lie is given to the implication that 'tobacco smoking kills' by the large numbers of relatively happy smokers who reach the age of average life expectancy in reasonable condition – saying, like Mark Twain, that reports of their death have been greatly exaggerated. It is also difficult to maintain that 'smoking leads to lung cancer' when nine out of ten smokers never get it.

There are 1.8 million smokers in Denmark. Each year 55,000 people die, 25,000 of them smokers; 3,200 deaths are due to lung cancer. If we accept the worst-case estimate that 80 per cent of the annual cases of lung cancer afflict smokers, then the figure is 2,400 out of the 25,000 smokers dead – less than one tenth. Finally, it is unlikely that those smokers who die from lung cancer have contracted it from their smoking. There are many other important factors that may cause lung cancer – the same ones, presumably, that cause the disease in non-smokers.

The inaccuracy of mortality statistics

Death certificates do not say whether people are smokers or non-smokers; the distinction is not usually made on hospital

Table 1: Post-mortem rates in different countries

Country	% of deaths occurring in hospital	% autopsy performed all ages	% autopsy performed age 65+
Austria	61	35	31
Denmark	56	32	c. 25
England & Wales	63	27	23
W. Germany	53	8	–
Ireland	62	7	4
Japan	67	4	3
Norway	73	16	c. 15
Sweden	79	37	36
Switzerland	54	19	16
USSR	24	31	–

Source: WHO, *World Health Statistics Annual* (1988)

charts. It is persistently repeated that 80 per cent of people who die of lung cancer are smokers. But this estimate is based on limited and uncertain material – estimated by people who need shock figures in their propaganda against tobacco smoking . . . and who are not entirely objective.

How accurate are mortality statistics? There are two problems. One is the accuracy of death certificates. The other is that post-mortems are the exception rather than the rule.

Britton found inconsistencies between clinicians' stated cause of death and autopsy diagnoses in as much as 65 per cent of cases. Many others found similar inconsistencies, and, in 1981, this led Cameron & McCoogan to contend that statistics based on death certificates cannot be valid.

Autopsies are performed in a minority of deaths. In Denmark it is under a third, in Japan it is only four per cent.

In the case of lung cancer, Feinstein & Wells found that of 654 autopsies where lung cancer *was* found, the diagnosis had not been made in over a third of the patients (37 per cent) while they were alive. Among non-smokers, there were 38 per cent undetected cases, among modest smokers 20 per cent, among moderate smokers 14 per cent, and among heavy smokers 10 to 11 per cent. They concluded that 'the more patients smoke, the greater the possibility that they have their lung cancer diagnosed before they die'. From this we might deduce that where an autopsy is *not* performed, unverified diagnoses of lung cancer will more often be made for smokers than for non-smokers. Moreover, as I mentioned earlier, there is the fact that 25 per cent of clinically discovered lung cancer turns out to be adenocarcinoma, which seldom starts in the lungs.

The possibility that secondary lung cancer (which begins in another organ) is diagnosed incorrectly as primary lung cancer (which begins in the lung) is not usually considered, because post-mortem analyses are carried out only when a death certificate is not routine, or when there is some other forensic reason. The most experienced histopathologist (specialist in diseased cell tissue) would hesitate to diagnose adenocarcinoma in the lung as primary, without excluding primary cancer in other organs (Faccini). This requires a detailed histological examination, which is seldom carried out.

When such cell-tissue investigations have been made, and the results compiled (Auerbach *et al.*), it is found that one-quarter (25 per cent) of the carcinomas are adenocarcinomas, almost all of them secondary. It is interesting that epidermoid cell tumours, which are usually a reaction to irritants such as asbestos, soot or tar, are found in about 35 per cent of the cases of lung cancer in smokers and almost never with non-smokers. In non-smokers adenocarcinomas account for 65 per cent of cases of lung cancer; in some studies up to 100 per cent (Wu). Therefore if passive smoking is responsible for lung cancer, it is odd that non-smokers mostly get adenocarcinomas and seldom epidermoid cancers.

We must also consider whether the increase in reported lung cancer deaths might be connected to improved diagnosis, as well as a greater focus on this problem in recent years. X-ray, bronchoscopy and tests for certain cells in saliva have become more common. So, the 'epidemic' could be more the result of medical progress than of changes in the incidence of the disease. We are looking more intensely for it, and we are more skilled in finding it.

So statistics quoted in the tobacco debate have to be taken with some caution. The majority of published papers may suggest that smokers have a higher risk of contracting lung cancer. But this must be proven before the allegation can be taken seriously and used as a basis for prohibitive legislation.

Cancer is not caused by smoking tobacco. When nine out of ten smokers never get lung cancer, smoking cannot be considered a sufficient cause. Other factors must play a role.

Since non-smokers also contract lung cancer, it is not necessary to smoke to get the disease. It has other causes, then. Since smoking is neither a necessary nor a sufficient cause, scientific theory maintains that causal connection cannot be made. Smoking may be a *contributory* factor in the development of lung cancer in certain cases – but that is very different from insisting that tobacco smoking inevitably leads to cancer. It may be that lung cancer is more likely if you smoke – but this also needs a proof beyond the epidemiological. That many observations point in this direction is still not sufficient to establish cause.

Risk assessment

The assertion must, therefore, be: smoking *may* lead to cancer. As sucking peppermints may also lead to cancer (this has never been proven, either, but swabbing rabbit ears with peppermint oil for ten years could easily lead to a cancerous reaction), the importance of the allegation must be evaluated by estimating the risk. If the risk of getting cancer from smoking happened to be of the same order as that of dying in a car accident, most people would ignore it. The common feeling among smokers is that the risk can be lived with, and many choose to do so.

Tobacco has never been documented as a cause of death – apart from those rare cases where children have eaten it. Tobacco smoking cannot be given as a cause of death on death certificates. In the Danish Health Department's mortality statistics, and in the international code for causes of death, there are no deaths due to tobacco smoking.

The diseases usually mentioned in connection with smoking are lung cancer and ischaemic heart failure (conditions resulting from a deficiency of blood supply to the heart muscles). Chronic obstructive lung diseases (such as emphysema), as well as bronchitis, asthma, thrombosis, arteriosclerosis and allergies, are also listed. The latter diseases are not deadly and do not have the same terrifying effect as lung cancer and heart failure, so they are not used in anti-smoking propaganda with the same intensity, although they cost far more in sick leave because of their greater frequency.

These 'tobacco-related' diseases amount to about 40 per cent of all deaths:

Lung cancer	6%
Ischaemic heart failure	28%
Chronic obstructive lung diseases	4%

with some others sharing the last few per cent.

It is difficult to differentiate between the potential causes, because we are exposed to a wide range of situations that might influence our health. It is rarely possible to make a convincing argument for ascribing responsibility to a particular factor in a specific disease. Insurance cases involving occupational injuries show how difficult it is prove in court that one definite activity is responsible for an injury or illness (whether disease or death).

Heart failure is traditionally associated with the hard-working businessman, with the inadequacies of missed or hasty meals, a lack of exercise, unsettling working conditions, interrupted sleep, and other indicators of a stressed life that include excessive tobacco smoking. If it is among people of this ilk (typically a majority of men) that most heart failure patients are found, then there will also be a majority of heavy smokers (and drinkers).

Other factors are clearly of greater significance than smoking in many cases. In respiratory diseases, for example, consider housing standards, working conditions (dust, solvents, cleaning liquids), diet, clothing, hygiene, physical condition, vitamin intake, social level, and cultural norms.

Allergies and tobacco

It is often suggested that allergies are caused by smoking and asthma is said to be aggravated by tobacco. Allergies are a reaction to a certain substance, the allergen. Tobacco allergy exists, as do allergies towards practically any substance, but it is extremely rare. When specialists search for the allergen in a particular case they run through an established list of sub- stances. Tobacco is placed very low on the list.

The nuisance value of tobacco smoke on allergic patients, especially asthmatics, is avidly studied, but the results do not confirm the allegation that smoking provokes asthmatic attacks. It is unclear how hypersensitivity to cat hairs or grass pollen could be influenced by tobacco. A number of asthma patients do report subjective inconvenience from a smoky atmosphere. Many other asthmatics, however, like to smoke, and do not report any inconvenience – some even maintain that they feel relief from their asthma by smoking. There are several papers showing that tobacco smoke has no negative effect on asthma patients, and that it does not increase the likelihood of attacks. It is true that other papers suggest the opposite, but it is almost impossible to correct these for subjective reactions. Asthmatic children, who have no preconceived opinions about tobacco, have remained in an atmosphere heavy with smoke without any subjective or objective aggravation being observed. The sugges- tion that the smoke particles themselves have a negative effect is contradicted by my own (and others') experience in the Thirties and Forties when we prescribed asthma cigarettes to prevent attacks – in the absence of more potent remedies. The cigarettes were smoked under a small improvised tent, and many found relief this way. That the active agent in these asthma cigarettes was stramonium is another matter.

If tobacco and tobacco smoke have a dangerous cancerous effect, the lips and oral cavity should be expected to show the greatest number of cancer cases, because the lips of the cigar smoker are in direct contact, often even moist contact, with the cigar for hours each day. Pipe smokers often mention that it 'bites' their tongues, when the condensation runs down the stem into the mouth. Of course, in all kinds of smoking, the mucous membrane of the mouth, throat and bronchial tubes are in contact with warm tobacco smoke when it is at its most concen- trated. But the most common cancers in the lung are in the alveolar epithelium or the bronchioles, the deepest parts of a lung – and furthest from the smoke. This is not what you would expect if smoke was the primary cause.

Cancer of the lips and oral cavity are given as the cause of seven deaths in Denmark in 1987 – out of 55,000; cancer of the tongue, 35 cases; cancer of the whole nasopharyngeal region, 224 cases (it is difficult to imagine tobacco smoke as a contributory factor in cancer of the roots of teeth, the maxillary sinuses, and the salivary glands); cancer of the windpipe and throat, 96 cases. But lung cancer deaths amount to 3,200 cases. These figures do not seem to confirm the carcinogenic effect of tobacco smoke; not even when we take into account that the cellular tissue varies in kind and in sensitivity between the regions mentioned, and that not all smokers inhale, so that the smoke comes in direct contact with the pulmonary mucous membrane.

Chronic bronchitis

It becomes more understandable if tobacco smoking is alleged to cause chronic bronchitis. Such a contention will be difficult to prove because much bronchitis is never treated, and therefore never registered, and because bronchitis varies greatly in severity. It is almost accepted – or used to be – as a concomitant of certain trades (asbestos workers, miners, grinders), certain social groups (slums), and certain age groups (babies and the elderly – the latter rather from bad circulation than from external factors). Chronic bronchitis is multi-factorial, which makes it extremely difficult to give relative weights to the potential factors – and almost impossible to quantify the degree to which tobacco smoking is responsible.

Lung cancer is, however, still the big issue in the controversy. According to accepted estimates, it takes about twenty years (the latent period) for a carcinogenic factor to result in clinical cancer. If smoking is a decisive factor, and if most smokers start smoking at the age of twenty, we should observe a steep increase in lung cancer among smokers from the age of forty. Between forty and fifty, according to the 1987 death statistics of the

Table 2: Deaths from lung cancer in Denmark (1987)

Age	Men	Women	Men + women combined	Cumulative total
15–19	–	1	1	1
20–24	–	–	0	1
25–29	–	1	1	2
30–34	6	0	6	8
35–39	14	9	23	31
40–44	30	17	47	78
45–49	46	33	79	157
50–54	103	65	168	325
55–59	169	132	301	686
60–64	314	162	476	1102
65–69	442	173	615	1717
70–74	435	177	612	2329
75–79	376	154	530	2859
80–84	204	76	280	3139
85+	91	45	136	3275
Total	2230	1045	–	–

Note: the right-hand column is the cumulative total for men and women up to that age. There is no marked increase until after the age of 55; note the many cases between ages 65 and 75.

Danish Health Department, 76 males and 50 females died of lung cancer. Whether they were smokers or not is not recorded. Between fifty and sixty, 272 and 197 respectively. Not until after the age of 60 is there a marked increase, following very precisely the increase in deaths from all other causes. This does not indicate a relationship with smoking – on the contrary.

It has never been demonstrated that tobacco smoking leads to cancer. Researchers have never succeeded in producing lung cancer in animal experiments, not even in guinea pigs living the majority of their lives in a highly concentrated tobacco atmosphere.

Nor has anyone identified patients with lung cancer who have been exposed solely to tobacco smoke – and no other pollutants whatsoever. It has, therefore, never been possible to ascertain the true responsibility of tobacco smoke in the development of lung cancer – the more so as lung cancer does occur in patients who have never been exposed to tobacco smoke.

Figure 1: Deaths from lung cancer in Denmark (1987)

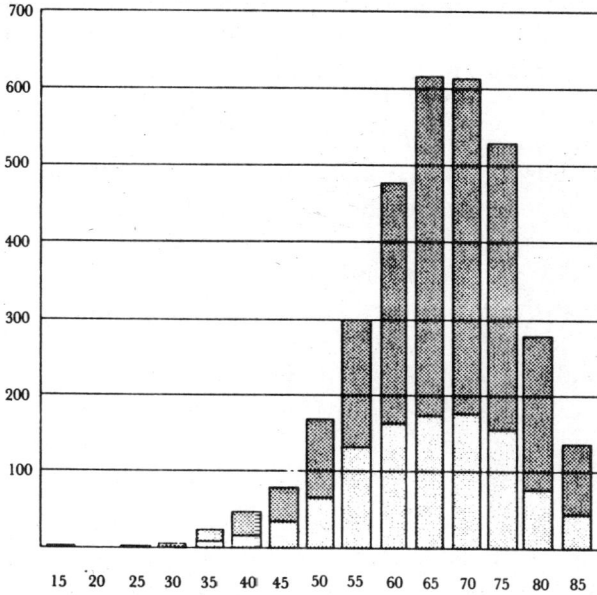

Note: the same data as in Table 2, presented as a bar-chart. Note the peak at average life expectancy. White bars = women; black bars = men

Figure 2: Deaths from lung cancer in Denmark (1987)

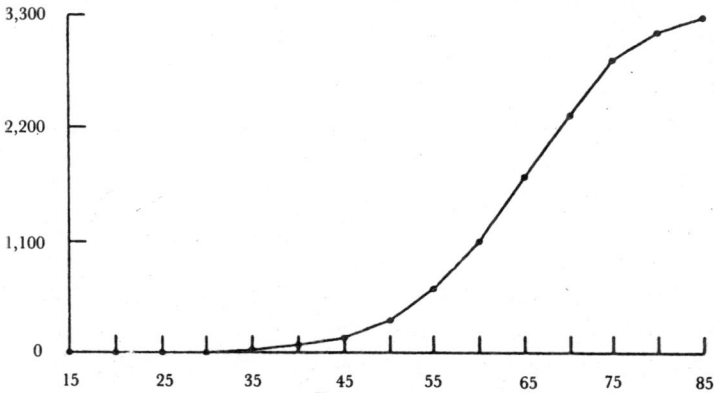

Note: the last column of Table 2, as a graph

The connection between smoking and lung cancer is statistical: there is a majority of smokers in a specific group, those dying of lung cancer. This is stated as a proof of causal connection, although there is no logical basis for it. The number of storks has decreased, the number of births has decreased, hence. . . . Coincidence is not causality.

The US Surgeon General, with the Royal College of Physicians in Great Britain and many other eminent scientific institutions, considers that these statistical coincidences are proofs of causality. This seems to have so impressed the world that the issue is now widely regarded as beyond discussion. It is on this basis that estimates are made showing that in the coming years so many millions or billions will 'die from tobacco smoking'. For example, at the 7th WHO Conference on Tobacco and Health in Perth, Australia, in April 1990, Dr Peto claimed that '250 million victims of tobacco will die in their prime of life (age thirty five to sixty-nine)': a scare story that was circulated in the world's press. The implication is that a similar number of lives will be spared if tobacco smoking is stopped altogether. The question is, for how long?

Cancer and heavy industry

As I have said, statistical coincidence is not proof of causal connection. Furthermore, there are many other papers offering statistics pointing in the opposite direction. For instance, there is the increasing lung cancer mortality among non-smokers, initially published in the United States in 1978 and since then in many other places in the world.

And there is the geographical distribution of lung cancer, which is unequal, concentrated in industrial areas, and which does not coincide with the geographical distribution of heavy smokers. (Fig. 3)

If lung cancer frequencies in various countries are compared, essential differences are found which cannot be explained by coincidental connection with tobacco smoking; many papers even show the opposite. In some countries, such as Austria, the frequency of lung cancer has been almost constant for the last few decades. Other countries, such as Japan, have had an increasing frequency of lung cancer from a very low starting point. In England and Wales lung cancer mortality was increasing, but is now decreasing. These variations do not relate to smoking habits in the respective countries. (Fig. 4)

In Japan, 85 per cent of all men smoke; and Japan has the world's lowest lung cancer mortality – 15 per 100,000 in the 1950s. But the younger generation – which has the same or lower tobacco consumption – shows a clear increase in lung cancer frequency, estimated at 100 per 100,000 by the end of this century. The increased frequency does not follow smoking habits, and a connection must be sought in other risk-creating conditions.

England and Wales, on the other hand, had quite a high frequency of lung cancer, increasing from 160 per 100,000 in the fifties to a maximum of 250 per 100,000 in 1970. Since then the figure has declined to 150. The increase in the number of lung cancer cases up to 1970 corresponded nicely to the increase in tobacco consumption (the latent period taken into account). But the fall in the following years has occurred, despite the fact that tobacco consumption has been the same – or rather has been increasing.

Austrian men show a rather high and constant lung cancer mortality, 160 out of 100,000 from the 1950s to the 1980s, compared to Japan (15 to 50 per 100,000 in the same period) – though the consumption of cigarettes is higher in Japan than in Austria.

In the same way, low lung cancer frequency has been shown (by Belcher 1987) in a group of women who have smoked more than any other group in the history of the UK. Increasing lung cancer frequency in a number of countries is based on increasing lung cancer frequency among non-smokers (Koo 1983, Hinds 1984, Anton-Culver 1988).

The United States and Canada have the highest *per capita* consumption of cigarettes in the world, but they are only listed as number 8 and 15 in regard to lung cancer mortality (males). On the other hand, Finland, England, and the Netherlands have lower cigarette consumption but higher lung cancer mortality.

Figure 3: Geographical incidence of deaths from lung cancer

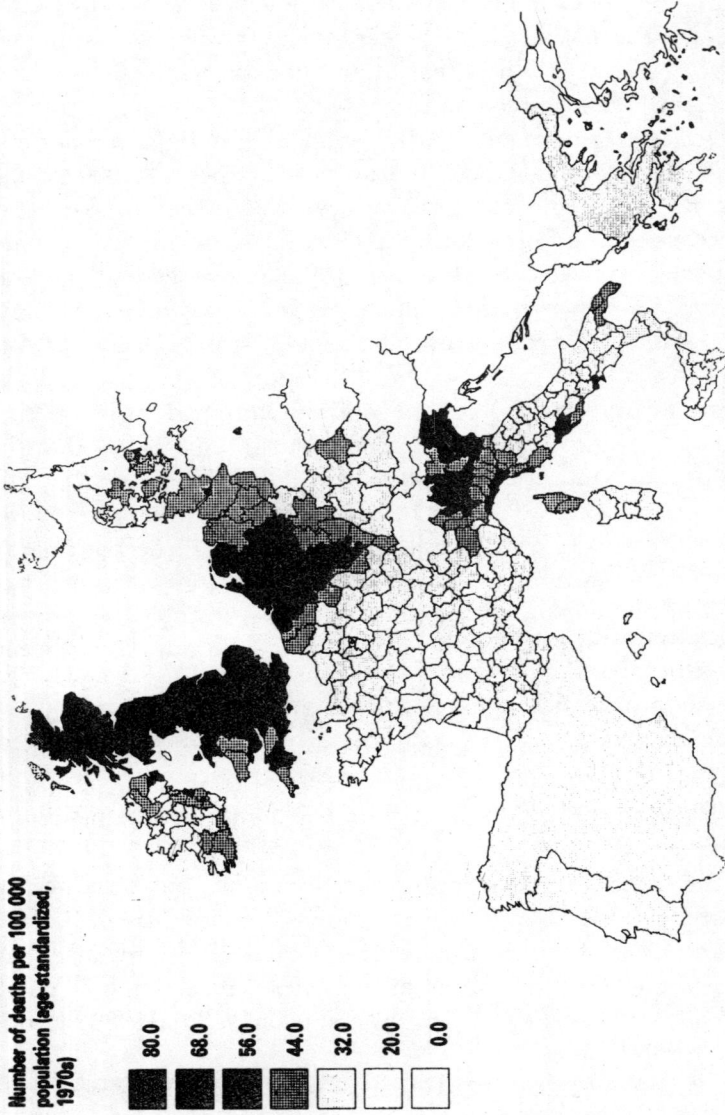

Number of deaths per 100 000 population (age-standardized, 1970s)

- 80.0
- 68.0
- 56.0
- 44.0
- 32.0
- 20.0
- 0.0

Source: Compiled for the European Commission by the International Agency for Research on Cancer

Figure 4: Lung cancer rates in England & Wales, and Japan

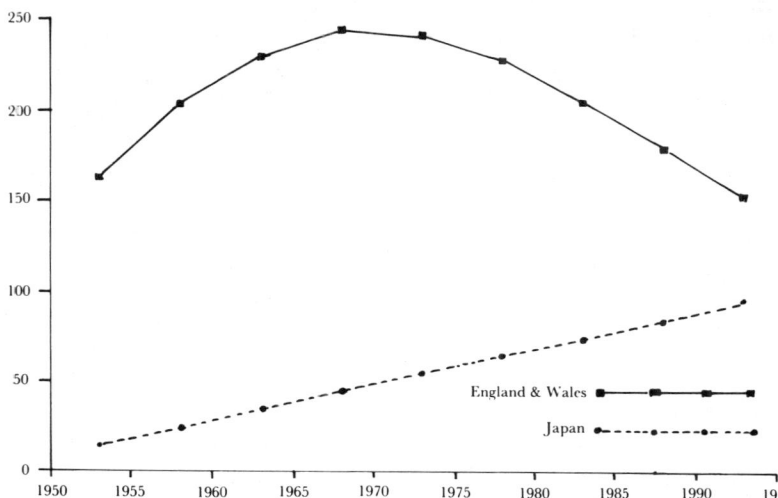

Note: observations made between 1953–83; 1988–93 predicted (rates are per 100,000 males aged 40–74)

These circumstances indicate that there are other, more positive, risk factors than smoking in developing lung cancer. In fact, they are evidence *against* such a connection.

The statistics used as a basis for the connection between smoking and lung cancer could be applied, more convincingly, to the connection with housing standards, food habits, working conditions, psychological constitution, or hereditary conditions ('cancer families'). Some British studies, for instance, show a greater relation between lung cancer and women's jobs than tobacco. Curiously, in recent years there has been shown a very strong correlation to association with pet birds. Pigeon breeders and cage-bird keepers have a higher than normal mortality from lung cancer.

If all these uncertainties are ignored an above-average mortality rate among smokers in the lung cancer group is observed, despite the difficulties of deciding who are smokers, who are not, and of quantifying the extent of smoking. The magical figure of 75 to 80 per cent keeps on appearing. Accepting this figure for the sake of argument, this means that 2,400 out of the 3,200 lung cancer deaths annually in Denmark are smokers, 800 are not. If the smokers did not smoke and were non-smokers, 25 per cent of them, 600, would still die of non-smoker lung cancer, which means that, even using the anti-smokers' dubious statistics, the number of deaths that could be ascribed to tobacco smoking could not be more than 1,800. And this should be reduced to 1,350 to account for the 25 per cent with adenocarcinoma. If we note that 1,100 are over 60 when they die, leaving 250 deaths a year (out of a total of 55,000) in 'the prime of life', then perhaps the problem is not so great that it justifies the intensity and bitterness of the attacks against smoking.

Using mortality figures, and estimating who were smokers and who were not, the ratio between smokers and non-smokers' death rates can be calculated for specific diseases. This will give a figure for the relative risk: it is 1.0 when the number of deaths in the two groups is equal, and so is the risk. Above 1.0 the risk is rising, below 1.0 it is diminishing. The Royal College of Physicians state in *Report on Smoking and Health 1971* that this rate is 10.8 for lung cancer, 1.7 for cardiovascular diseases. (Others give different ratios.) The interesting thing is, however, that the death rate can be below 1.0 for certain diseases, which means that smokers more rarely die from the disease in question. This has been found by, for example, Kahn – 0.9 for cancer of the rectum, and Hammond – 0.78 and 0.66 for cancer of the colon among smoking and heavily smoking women, respectively. Others have found a low ratio for tumours in the central nervous system. In the case of Parkinson's disease the ratio is as low as 0.26, as it has been found that 70 per cent of a group of patients with Parkinsonism had never smoked. Similar observations have been made concerning trigeminal neuralgia and diabetes, which apparently attacked smokers more rarely than non-smokers.

But I do not suppose that anybody will recommend the absurd consequence of smoking tobacco to reduce the risk of getting these diseases: nor that they will recommend you quit smoking in order not to get any of the others. Causality does not necessarily have anything to do with one's place in the respective risk groups. If any of this really did hold good, we could choose whether to have cancer in the lungs or the intestines . . . by smoking – or abstaining from it.

The other group of diseases in which excess mortality among smokers is perceived is the cardiovascular. The claimed excess mortality is far lower here, almost down to the statistical level where it cannot be considered as proven. On the other hand, we are talking here about a far larger group of patients.

Once again diagnosis is a minefield of inexactitude. Heart diseases are a diagnostical mess and there is no doubt that many deaths are simply reported as heart failure without detailed investigation. The diagnosis of heart death is arbitrary and not a good basis for viable statistics.

There are the same uncertainties and confounding factors with heart death as there are for the rest of the 'tobacco-related' causes of death. If lung cancer is multi-factorial, this is even truer for heart diseases. One set of heart diseases have definitely nothing to do with tobacco. This is true for rheumatic fever, damage after infections, such as children's diseases, and specific infections affecting the heart proper and its valve system. The overdeveloped heart, 'athletic heart', that has been trained for peak performance, ages more rapidly and is more likely to suffer ischaemia.

It is principally 'the ischaemic heart' – the heart that is undersupplied with blood because its arterial system is constricted by sclerosis or the like – which is the most frequent reason for angina pectoris, circulation failure, and heart failure, and which is the most frequent cause of death in all developed countries.

Curiouser and curiouser . . .

The US Surgeon General and others have, over the years, confirmed their opinion that there is a connection between these diseases and tobacco smoking – repeated so often and with so much authority that it has become a dogma. The Framingham Heart Study, the largest and most meticulous on this subject, finds that ex-smokers have fewer heart diseases than continuing smokers, but also that they have fewer heart diseases than people who have never smoked, and for that matter finds no significant relation between smoking and heart diseases. A great number of scientific and medical authorities, even the Royal College of Physicians (1983), noticed the striking difference in the frequency of heart diseases in different countries, quite independent of smoking habits. WHO's large MONICA programme (Monitoring of Cardiovascular Disease), which is now in its fifth year, and which has registered 15 million people in 26 countries, finds no connection so far between heart death and known risk factors (smoking, increased blood pressure, increased cholesterol, excess weight). Other studies find that, for instance, lowering of blood pressure leads to a clearly decreased risk of heart disease. It is, nonetheless, interesting that the so-called 'multiple risk factor intervention trials', attempts to alter people's lifestyles and get them to 'live a healthy life', have given barely significant results. This should give anti-smokers pause for thought . . . and give obsessive legislators cause for hesitation.

The US Surgeon General's assertions are at odds with the Framingham findings. The group of heart diseases that may have something to do with tobacco smoking may also be caused by other and well-known conditions: increased cholesterol, excess weight, and increased blood pressure. The later death comes the more difficult it is to identify the correlations. At any rate, only a minority of heart deaths show one and only one cause of the disease. In all probability there is a degree of interaction between all these factors. But to what extent?

Bacon and beans

Is it twice as dangerous for a bacon consumer to smoke tobacco than it is for a bean eater? Or has tobacco smoking the opposite effect, so that the effect of the pork fat is diminished or perhaps even abolished? Green et al. (1986) find that smokers rarely develop increased blood pressure. Pharmacologists work consciously and directly with the interaction of substances. Many composite medications are directly aimed at such interaction. If it is an error to give morphine to a person under the influence of alcohol, it is because the effects not only add up but are dangerously intensified – synergistic. And when drunks are given coffee, as a stimulant, it is in the hope that the caffeine will limit the effect of the alcohol. When it is a question of the influence of substances on the heart, especially their liability in the development of ischaemic heart disease, such considerations are not mentioned. Tobacco is dangerous. Cholesterol is dangerous, alcohol is dangerous. Great efforts are made to assess the danger of these substances. But how they interact is obviously of no interest to anybody. Might it be that the damaging effect of tobacco on the heart is neutralized by a suitable amount of alcohol? Or that tobacco neutralizes the effect of increased cholesterol . . .?

One of the few allegations about the effects of smoking on health that seems to be universally accepted is on the birth weight of children born to smoking mothers (although the evidence has never been convincingly corrected for confounding factors, especially social conditions).

Smoking mothers do, however, according to many studies, bear children with a birth weight 200 to 300g lower than average – an argument against tobacco smoking that is made with conviction. The argument, though, assumes a high birth weight is a positive attribute. Nobody can prove that children with a birth weight of 3kg have a poorer start in life than children weighing 3.25kg at birth. Even premature babies weighing only 2kg grow into fully viable individuals when given skilful care, and they manage to be just as robust as full-term babies. Social and psychological conditions have a rather more decisive influence on children's birth weight (Zachau-Christiansen).

Is a birth weight of 5kg invariably better than one of 4kg – or 3kg? No. The most frequent birth defects and many complications at the birth itself are, in affluent societies, caused by babies that are too big: the size of the head is especially significant for the course of the birth. So it would not necessarily be a bad thing if the average birth weight was 300g lower. The difficulty in recommending pregnant women to smoke tobacco is that it has never been demonstrated how much they have to smoke to

produce the stated effect. Once again, there is only a rough
distinction between smokers and non-smokers. One must ask: Is
a smoker one who smokes one daily cigarette, or six, or twenty,
or thirty? Is there no distinction between dose and effect? No one
admits it. But smoking has to be condemned, under all circumstances! If you have a history of small children it would be
sensible to abstain from smoking during pregnancy. But the
converse cannot be advised – solely on moral grounds. Because
nobody is interested in talking about dependence on dosage. It
has to be all or nothing. 'All' is treated as though it were sixty a
day – so it has to be nothing. But what about five a day?

If care for the health of pregnant women and the well-being of
unborn children were really on the minds of the establishment, it
would be easy to use what we already know about the ideal
conditions for a successful pregnancy and a healthy childhood.
Reinforced by Zachau-Christiansen's study, among others, we
would see to it that pregnant women had decent housing, sufficient food, a reasonable income, and non-stressful work. We
content ourselves with concern over smoking habits.

One harmful effect can be maintained beyond all discussion:
the financial one. Tobacco has gradually become rather expensive, thanks to heavy taxation, and many people quit smoking because they perceive the cost as too high in proportion to
the pleasure. It is true that doctors visit homes where everything
has been neglected and the food cupboard is empty, while
cigarette butts lie everywhere. People are sometimes so desperate
that common sense goes out of the window and the choice
between options no longer exists. Even here the causal connection is unclear. The moralist will maintain that the misery is due
to tobacco – the more understanding person that smoking is the
last consolation of the miserable.

It is not generally held that non-smokers are healthier, or
happier, or richer than smokers. It has never been proven that
the finances of non-smokers are better, or that the smokers' vice
results in poverty. This could be related to the thought that the
sum of the cost of vices might always be constant, and that he
who does not smoke often does something else. Very little of
what is fun in this world is free.

4
The Beneficial Effects of Smoking

In 1748 Holberg had already noticed the positive effects of smoking. In his *Epistle to Collegium Politicum*, he takes a look at pleasures previously considered harmless and even useful, and satirizes the way respectable men had attacked dancing and the theatre, finding them pernicious and harmful. Holberg takes as his example the phenomenon of 'daily smoking tobacco'.

He writes: 'After having smoked a couple of pipes of tobacco, which do give ideas for projects and fill up the brain with all kinds of concepts, and thereby having pondered this question and considered everything that can be said *pro et contra* concerning this matter . . .', and continues with a condemnation of the 'scandalous vice of tobacco smoking', with all the ironical citizen's indignation that the old parodist could mobilize. It is priceless fun, especially in the light of most comments against tobacco in today's debate.

Stimulant?

Holberg was aware of the positive aspects of smoking, although not unconditionally. But his early observations of the impact on perception, association, concentration, and intellectual performance have been corroborated in our time in many publications reporting the results of psychological, psychotechnical, physiological, neuroelectrical, neurochemical, and pharmacological tests. I refer at random to a number of these works, and also to reviews (with vast references to the literature), such as Warburton's 'The puzzle of nicotine use' in M. Lader's *The Psychopharma-*

cology of Addiction, or Wald & Froggatt's *Nicotine, Smoking, and the Low Tar Programme*.

Experimental studies show that smoking tobacco is followed by stimulation of the nervous system, centrally as well as peripherally, intellectually as well as emotionally. Smoking makes one cleverer, more efficient, brighter, more balanced, more harmonious, and more at ease. These are all wonderful statements for a smoker on the defensive.

Social mediator?

To this can be added unscientific testimony about smoking as a catalyst for social contact, as a provider of opportunities for contact, as a solace in distress, as a stimulator of thought. Smoking as a stimulant in a wider sense seems doubtful to me, and apart from the appetite-suppressant effect, the stimulating aspect is probably questionable.

In brief, it can be said that tobacco smoking is an enhancement of the quality of life for many people: it tastes good, it increases our well-being in many situations, it is a ritual act that helps us pace our day and sweeten it. Negative things could be said about waste of time and affectation in relation to five o'clock tea, but it has, indeed, contributed morally and practically to Great Britain's ability to survive ordeals. The tradition of a drink before dinner can be criticized, but the relaxation and contact that it promotes, besides stimulating the expectation of the meal, have their positive aspects. The reasonably arranged beer break surely has alleviated much physical drudgery. But all these social traditions contain the possibility of running to excess and losing control, if one steps outside the formal rituals. The same can be said about smoking tobacco. If it was always controlled by a set of norms, we would hardly have got this hysterical about it. Too little and too much. . . . How harmful is five o'clock tea, one could ask?

There are several positive qualities in smoking tobacco. It can hardly be maintained that smoking is healthy – but should one ignore the value of having a break, reflecting, taking a rest,

Figure 5:   Ideal weight related to smoking

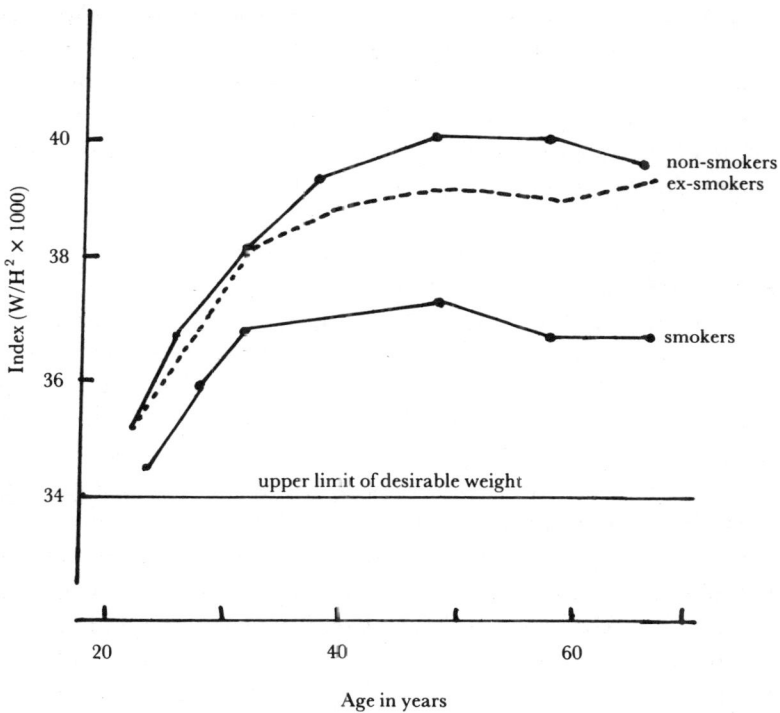

Note: the body-weight of smokers (as an index related to age and
height) is closer to the ideal weight than that of ex- and non-
smokers (*Source*: Rudman 1987)

enjoying the company of others? Should one ignore the unhealthy aspect of having to abstain from something one likes to
do and finds pleasure in . . .?

Some diseases DON'T attack smokers

These reflections are given a greater impetus by another
thought. I mentioned that smokers are less likely than non-
smokers to contract intestinal cancer, Parkinson's disease,

trigeminal neuralgia, tumours in the central nervous system, and diabetes. It should not be construed from these positive intimations that non-smoking causes these conditions (remember our reservations about epidemiological demonstrations of causal connections), nor that brain tumours could be prevented by heavy cigarette smoking.

Part of the paradox is that miners and asbestos workers who smoke contract lung injuries and lung cancer less often than their non-smoking colleagues. One theory is that smoking stimulates the epithelial cilia[1], so that they are more active in transporting phlegm and dust out of the lung.

In quite a different context a definite improvement in the condition of senile dementia and Parkinsonism patients has been observed from tobacco smoking (or taking nicotine tablets).

Nor must we forget the many papers showing that performance decreases in a number of areas when smokers stop smoking. Ex-smokers tend to put on weight. Non-smokers are usually heavier than smokers. But don't change the habits of lifetime just yet: we still do not know which factor gives the greater risk of premature heart failure: heavy smoking or being overweight.

And what we miss the most is an investigation of how risky the worrying is!

---

1. Cilia: hair-like appendages on the cells that line the mucous membranes of the lung, passing particles along with a wave-motion (*Ed.*)

5

Definition of a Smoker

Every year, the Danish Health Department publishes its mortality statistics based on the previous year's recorded data: numbers, causes, gender, age, housing conditions, and so on. Whether the deceased smoked or not is not recorded and can only be discovered by asking after the event. Few hospital charts give information about smoking habits – indeed, for most people there are no charts at all. The deceased cannot answer, so we have to ask relatives, whose answers may not be reliable and may be affected by the bereavement, by fears over insurance, by the desire to tell the doctor what he wants to hear.

This results in a considerable uncertainty. More problems come from having to make such inquiries on a selected sample. The reliability of such research depends, among other things, upon how random the selection is. There will always be doubts about how representative such research actually is.

There is yet another uncertainty: that of describing deceased persons as 'smokers' or 'non-smokers'. When did smoking start or end, how much was smoked, when and for how long? Was he or she a heavy smoker, a casual smoker, smoker of what forms of tobacco? Did he or she inhale or not? All this is essential information for an assessment of the possible influence of smoking on the course of life or disease. The more detailed the questions, the more uncertain is the reliability of the answers.

One problem is that a substantial definition of a smoker is missing. A lady who, after retirement, starts smoking a cheroot with her evening coffee is from a moral point of view not a non-smoker. But a clinical assessment would consider her a non-smoker. In estimates of the possible harmful effects of tobacco, it would be absurd to place her in the same risk group as people who have inhaled 60 cigarettes daily since their school days. But this is precisely what has been done in the WHO's MONICA research and in many other papers.

But how do we define and subdivide a particular study group? How do we fix the limits? For the anti-smokers it is quite simple: everybody who smokes, no matter how much or how little, is made the target of the same campaign: smoking is harmful! There is no word of mitigation or doubt about the validity of this allegation.

It is precisely because the possible harmful effects of smoking are so inadequately explained that difficulties arise concerning the definition of sub-groups. People don't always divide easily into smokers and non-smokers: the whole gradation of smoking becomes unclear. There will be people who throughout their lives have a highly varied consumption, in some periods smoking heavily, in others not at all. How do we place them? If you stop at the age of forty, what are you at the age of sixty, smoker or non-smoker? We may create a group called ex-smokers, but does that make any sense? Does this have any value if the group cannot clearly demonstrate a better health status and survival rate than those who have kept on smoking?

If statistics showing causes of death are going to be our basis, then the exactness of the information from relatives is going to be critical. 'He did stop, I think, when he retired . . .' 'Well, he seemed to be hale and hearty, I believe. Perhaps he coughed a bit in the morning . . .' If we can't use the cause-of-death statistics, what then – if the non-smoker group do not declare themselves healthy, happy, and well, compared to the smoker group? And if they do, on what objective criteria? How is health measured, how is the quality of life measured?

As long as the threshold values for tobacco smoking – the amount that has to be smoked to harm the most sensitive tissues – are not known, humanity cannot be divided into the two groups, smokers and non-smokers. The clinician, the hygienist, and the toxicologist would be interested in finding such threshold values and being able to give qualified statements about tobacco smoking.

The statistics will continue to be distorted as long as moderate smokers (those whose consumption is below the as-yet-unknown threshold values) are included as smokers. As far as their health is concerned, they will be like non-smokers but count as smokers, and so their health will blur and dilute the possible damage caused by heavy smoking.

The MONICA project has a category of 'regular smokers' – characterized by smoking 1 gram of pipe tobacco or at least one cigar per week! One must question the scientific sense in expecting to be able to appreciate differences of medical consequence between one cigar per week and none at all.

On the other hand, the propaganda of the anti-smokers will be impeded if they have to accept moderate smoking as unharmful and limit their campaign to major consumption only. What they may gain in credibility they will lose in support from the fanatical tobacco-haters who, in spite of the facts, want to condemn tobacco smoking to any extent and under all circumstances. The whole crusade against tobacco smoking would lose its punch.

6

The Teachings of Paracelsus

'Tobacco contains 100 dangerous substances', 'Tobacco smoking leads to cancer', 'Tobacco destroys your health'. The statements are diverse and unsubtle. Whether they are right or wrong can only be determined when we are talking about tangible quantities, specific concentrations of substances. If this is not done, anything could replace tobacco. Salt destroys your health. Bread contains 100 dangerous substances. TV screens lead to cancer. . . .

As early as the sixteenth century, Paracelsus taught us that there are no poisonous substances, only incorrect dosages. This seems to have been forgotten in the current debate. Poisonous or not poisonous, this depends solely on dosage. And without stating what doses of which substances we are talking about, the question is meaningless.

This means that in the tobacco debate we need to investigate the content of tobacco and tobacco smoke, find out how the constituents are set free, and what their effects are, in what concentration, on the affected tissue. We need to ascertain how respective tissues will react against the substances in question in actual concentrations. It might be interesting to know that swabbing tar on shaved mouse bellies over a long period may cause skin cancers to develop. But it gives no real basis for assessing the effect of tobacco tar on pulmonary mucous membranes. The question here is: what is the effect of how much tar over how long a period of time? It has been estimated that the effect of the tar on mouse bellies is equivalent to the effect on lung tissue of 1,000 cigarettes smoked daily over fifty years.

As Paracelsus teaches us, neither strychnine, potassium

65

cyanide, nor fly agaric[1] are poisonous as long as the doses are sufficiently small. We recognize in daily life that there are threshold values below which any substance is harmless to the organism. Even the anti-alcohol lobby promotes threshold values. There are different threshold values for different organisms. What is fatal to one kind of tissue may be harmless to another. This is true not only for poisons, but also for cold, warmth, radiation, and so on.

Well, what about the substances liberated through smoking?

Hundreds of different chemical compounds released by the smoking of tobacco can be isolated and analyzed – as many as 3,200 substances have been noted. Most of them are present in the smoke in such tiny quantities that they are well below the existing threshold values and are harmless.

So, although it is correct that tobacco contains a number of poisonous substances, it is, however, of no immediate importance for the debate because of the low doses. A cigar weighing 5 grams contains 1 to 3 per cent nicotine, about 100 milligrams, more than double the lethal dosage, enough to kill anybody who eats it. But cigars are normally not eaten, and should not be eaten. The maximum quantities of nicotine absorbed from a cigar by smoking are far below the threshold value.

In pharmacology a certain therapeutic dosage is recommended for each medicament; the dosage which gives the wanted effect. A maximum dosage is also defined, which is the one you can justifiably administer without hurting the patient. Finally, a lethal dosage is stated, which is the smallest dosage necessary to threaten the patient's life. It is characteristic that the therapeutic dosage is a one-time dosage, and that the time span of the effect is known, which means the time to wait before a new dose can be administered. Doses and maximum doses may also be listed on a twenty-four hour basis, while lethal dosage (which is usually ten times as much as maximum dosage) is considered a one-time dosage. This means that when therapeutic

---

1. The poisonous mushroom *Amanita muscaria*, once used as an intoxicant by peasants in Siberia and as a murder weapon by Dorothy L. Sayers. It also kills flies, hence the common name. (*Ed.*)

doses are given over several days, the lethal dosage may very well have been exceeded without doing any harm.

This is due to the decomposition and elimination of the substance, which means that the substance can be taken at certain intervals without critical concentrations being reached in the organism. You can have twenty alcoholic drinks[2] every day for years without any demonstrable tissue damage or intoxication. They just have to be distributed equally over twenty-four hours. The alcohol of one drink is metabolized and inactivated in seventy-five minutes, so you do not build up to significant alcohol levels at any time if you wait an hour and fifteen minutes before the next drink. (Alcohol was used in this way as treatment before the discovery of insulin, to nourish diabetic patients so that their sugar balance was not affected – as far as I know without damage to health). It is quite another matter if you have the twenty drinks at once. Then you probably drop dead, paralyzed by acute alcohol poisoning with sky-high blood levels.

As far as acute effects are concerned, we may talk about thresholds, as a matter of course. As to long-term effects, what doses over how long a period must be given? In the tobacco debate acute effects are of less interest than long-term effects; with lung cancer, the interest lies in consumption over twenty years.

Intensive smoking of a certain amount of tobacco can make you 'green' – with nausea, not envy – while the same amount or a larger quantity over a longer period has no noticeable effect whatsoever. This works in the same way as that described for alcohol. The alien substance is decomposed and eliminated, nicotine even more rapidly than alcohol (the time to cut the blood level by half is only half an hour). When assessing the effect of a substance at different doses, the time factor – the pace – of the smoking can be more important than the sheer number of smoked units. But this is totally ignored in the debate.

If decomposition and elimination of a substance are slower than absorption of it, it will accumulate, so despite intake of

2. 'Drink' means the small standard unit (14 ml of neat alcohol) as used by health advisors: a small whisky, a half pint of beer, a glass of wine, etc. (*Ed.*)

modest quantities, considerable concentrations can be found in the organism.

Accumulation in the tissues occurs with heavy metals. Even though the assimilated quantities are small, almost no elimination occurs. The substances accumulate in the organism, usually in specific tissues, where over the years they reach critical threshold values, poisoning and destroying the tissue. Lead and mercury are well-known sources of poisoning in certain regions; strontium 90 from radioactive fallout replaces calcium in bone tissue and emits damaging radiation from within. Fortunately, nicotine is rapidly eliminated and so does not accumulate; substances from the tar component in tobacco smoke may be identified in the tissues, but they have to be isolated from the host of similar substances (some produced by non-tobacco combustion, others in dust, and so on) that modern man inhales throughout his life. The components of tar are claimed to be associated with the cancerous effect on lungs. So we must eliminate *all* the potential sources, if possible. The frequency of lung cancer in those areas that were once heavily industrialized tells a very clear story.

In considering the precautions to be taken against pollution-related problems, WHO has sought to establish intake limits for a range of substances that may have a poisonous effect. This toxicological assessment has led to a list of admissible weekly intakes of these substances, a so-called TWI-value. The TWI-value is 'the quantity of a substance, which a human being, according to calculations and their preconditions, should be able to take in every week throughout their lives without any risk of damaging effects, and which at times might well be exceeded without having any health-related significance'. This seems to be a tolerant approach towards environmental pollution. But TWI values for tobacco smoking have not been established. The policy of WHO towards tobacco ignores such quantities. It maintains that tobacco smoking is harmful – in any quantity. Paracelsus seems to have spoken in vain here.

The effect with which the tobacco debate is most preoccupied is the carcinogenic effect, the susceptibility to cancer. All tissues are exposed to irritants throughout life, and the indications are that as long as these quantities and levels do not exceed certain limits, nothing will happen. Some of the components of tar are capable of provoking tumour cell growth. It is therefore clearly of specific interest to be able to measure such effects. But when it is at all possible (in mouse bellies), it is only at outrageous levels which are virtually impossible in daily life.

Where are the threshold values? How much are you supposed to smoke for how long to be at increased risk? Because the tissue reaction does not set in until after twenty years, assessing the connection between dose and effect becomes difficult.

Does a tissue 'remember' irritants? If so, for how long does it remember? At least twenty years – or what . . .? Will cigarettes smoked at puberty have an accumulating effect, which may harm you when you reach the average lifespan of seventy-four years? Or is the folly of youth mercifully forgotten, so that the converted ex-smoker, who quits his heavy consumption at the age of fifty, becomes as good as any non-smoker twenty years later? Much research has gone into these relationships, especially in connection with heart diseases. And despite the shock/horror propaganda claiming that you destroy your tissues, increase the risk and decrease your survival prospects, the moralist conclusion is that it is never too late to repent. This is corroborated with several epidemiological papers showing how much better and longer a new ex-smoker survives.

All these epidemiological studies suffer from the usual weaknesses, that they are entirely based on the credibility of the interview technique, the audacity with which the material is processed mathematically, and conclusions drawn from the calculations. These circumstances seem very much like the weather forecasts of the meteorologists, and deserve the same respect.

Physiological threshold values seem to be quite essential. Very little is known about them; so the assertions are much more extravagant. Nobody knows whether the harmful effect is proportional to the quantity of inhaled smoke (Figure 8, curve a), or if there is an intensified effect, so that the harmful effect is increased and the last one of 20 cigarettes is twice as harmful as the first one (curve c). Or perhaps the other way round: that the first one is the most dangerous, and that the harmful effect

Figure 6:   Some hypothetical curves

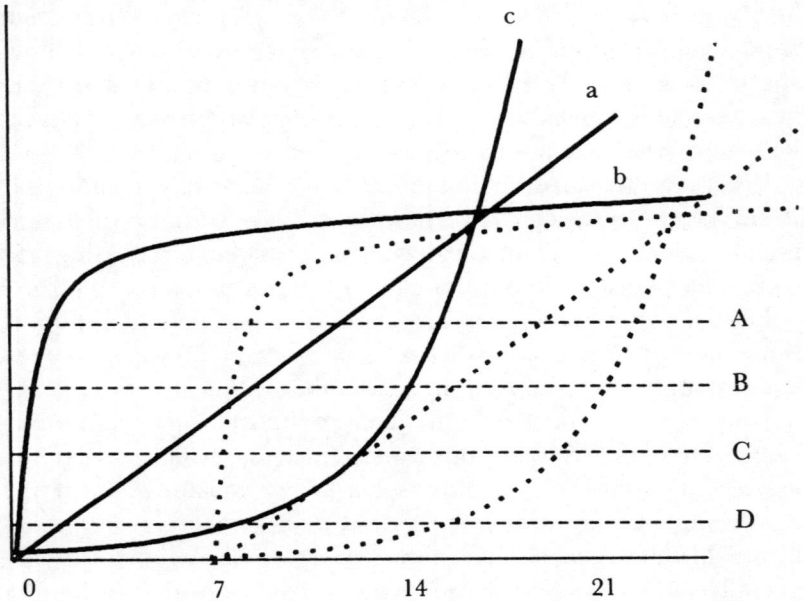

The vertical scale is an arbitrary and unknown unit of damage; the horizontal scale is the number of cigarettes smoked. No thresholds have been demonstrated. The curves are hypothetical: (a) a direct relationship between the damage sustained and the number of cigarettes smoked; (b) the relationship if it is the first few cigarettes that cause most damage; (c) the relationship if it is the last few. (A) is the threshold for the immediate effect of nicotine; (B) of tar; (C) for carbon monoxide over 10 years; (D) for carbon monoxide over 20 years.

decreases, so that the difference between cigarettes 19 and 20 can hardly be measured (curve b). Or can it be considered harmless to smoke less than a certain number, so that you may stay below a threshold value? That, say, seven daily cigarettes cannot be demonstrated as harmful, while the eighth is fatal . . . (the dotted curves). Nothing like this has ever been measured and until now there has been nothing scientifically tenable to give us clues to a solution to the problem: there exists no well-defined measure for the harmfulness of smoking.

   If threshold values were used, how should they be established?

The number of cigarettes smoked would not necessarily be a useful unit of measurement. Ten cigarettes smoked in an hour and a half might very well take you over some critical limit, which twenty cigarettes smoked in fourteen hours would not even touch. Ten cigarettes smoked in the open air will surely not be as harmful as the same number of cigarettes smoked in a narrow, badly ventilated room. Would the same quantity of tobacco smoke harm a person who breathes 10 cubic metres of indoor air in a certain time as much as one who gets through 200 cubic metres of fresh country air with exercise during the same period of time? Why always talk about the harmful effect in relation only to the daily number of cigarettes? How, then, may the extent of smoking be measured? The problem is still unsolved.

There are no means by which we can measure how prone a tissue is to develop a cancer; we have to await the first symptoms. One of the difficulties of this lies in the fact that many people develop pre-cancerous stages or manifest cancer which is not discovered until autopsy. As I repeat, only a minority are autopsied anyway.

So if we want to study the damage done to, say, people aged fifty by tobacco smoking, we have only statistics to work from. This means the number of lung cancer deaths in this age group distributed between smokers and non-smokers. In Denmark this amounts to less than ten cases. It is self-evident that selection into groups with different tobacco consumption will result in such small numbers that they are statistically unreliable. It would be frivolous from this material to make any judgements about the risk. It would also be true to say that those who die at the age of fifty cannot be statistically normal from a health point of view, and not comparable with the rest of the population.

This means that a population consisting of a one-year age group (in Denmark 70,000 50-year-old individuals) cannot give any valid result.

If the frequency of lung cancer in the whole population was ten per 100,000 then 10 per cent more deaths would mean one more, eleven per 100,000. And an increase in lung cancer deaths of 30 per cent would mean three more, thirteen per 100,000. To demonstrate something that looks like a statistical proof, we need a cohort at least ten times larger: around 1 million smokers, and preferably 1 million non-smokers as controls (which is to opt for the average population which, of course, comprises smokers as well as non-smokers). It would be quite an ambitious enterprise, which in Denmark would have to encompass all those born over a period of thirty years.

We here face the problem of whether to choose younger year groups with almost no cases of lung cancer or elderly groups with more cases. The results will be based solely on our choice. If we choose elderly groups, the consumption patterns will be unclear and difficult to clarify, and other factors simultaneously have greater influence. Many people have stopped smoking at various points in time after having smoked a varying number of cigarettes. How are pipe smokers and cigar smokers to be placed in relation to these, and how is their consumption to be made comparable? How about those who after a puritanical youth start smoking at a mature age . . .? The observations will also be blurred by the fact that after the age of sixty the normal death rate starts increasing – for all sorts of reasons. That means that lung cancer, as it were, is overlapped or overtaken by a number of other diseases as cause of death. To put it another way, other causes of death upset our observations of lung cancer, because those expected to die from 'tobacco related diseases', die of something else before that. It remains difficult to relate lung cancer to tobacco smoking.

Nobody knows anything about threshold values for the damaging effects of tobacco – nobody contemplates them. There is loose talk about smokers, non-smokers, heavy smokers (differently estimated by some at 15 cigarettes a day, by others at 20 cigarettes a day, and by still others at 30 a day), but never about the durability of smoking, and nothing at all about its time interval in the life process. That nobody can give the threshold values is one thing. But that nobody misses them betrays a deplorable level of scientific understanding – we have not taken to heart Paracelsus' lesson about dependence on dosage.

The controversy over the possible harmful effects of tobacco does not depend on correlations and facts. Anti-smokers seek to generate a general attitude by selective argument, spurning evidence that is awkward. This is what makes it so unintelligent and uninteresting. That such a level of argument occurs in our living rooms and in the press is understandable. But that the debate among physicians and scientists is at such a level is shameful.

Does this suggest that professional pundits push themselves forward in the tobacco debate for demagogical reasons? If so, what are their motives? Those who take part are few – and arrogant. The majority of professionals and medical authorities are totally uninvolved in these unessential problems. Tobacco and health – good Lord, there are much weightier threats against well-being and health. This is Per Degn and Erasmus Montanus crowing on the dunghill[3] – if those poseurs are not reconciled, let them bicker. The press enjoys it.

From where governments and the authorities, the EC, and WHO get their evidence remains obscure. And so do their arguments.

---

3. This is a reference to a famous – in Denmark – Holberg play *Erasmus Montanus* in which the eponymous hero starts as a peasant, becomes a student of philosophy, and – like so many of his kind – loses touch with reality. Per Degn is the old Dean of Philosophy who, perhaps senile, defends his wisdom and dignity. The pair have absurd discussions in nonsense rhymes. Definitely an anti-establishment work! (*Ed.*)

7

Which Substances have What Impact?

On this subject, the debate about the harmfulness of tobacco
smoking is very disorganized. Most of the discussion concerns
the creation of dependence, carcinogenic properties, poisoning,
and effects on the heart; and nobody can say precisely which
effects are due to what substances. If it was about the general
harmfulness of smoking, specificity might be irrelevant, but
there is a constant focusing on specific substances.

At times, carbon monoxide is the bogyman. At other times it is
nicotine. Neither of these would increase the risk of lung cancer
(although some reaction products from nicotine are suspected by
some researchers to be carcinogenic). Inhalation of smoke particles and tar substances is another matter. On the other hand,
they – tar and smoke particles – do not contribute to the pharmacological effect that keeps the 'tobacco slaves addicted to their
vice'. There is at the moment a lively debate about the sense or
non-sense in launching low-nicotine cigarettes. If, as it is
claimed, they enticed smokers to smoke more cigarettes, the
smokers would inhale more tar, which would be more likely to
give them lung cancer. Nicotine and tar content divides the
guardians and the lawyers into passionate groups who indulge in
intense debate on the basis of chemical and psychological research.

The physiologically interesting substances in the inhaled
smoke are nicotine, carbon monoxide (which is not present in the
tobacco, but is a result of the combustion process, as it is during
the combustion of all other substances), as well as tar substances
and smoke particles.

Roughly speaking, the assertions are that nicotine is the

poison; carbon monoxide has a harmful effect on the cardiovascular system; and tar increases the cancer risk. Other
effects are mentioned, but they are only given slight attention in
the debate compared to these which are the principal charges.
Many of the effects reported are ephemeral, and sooner or later
they are removed from the repertoire – either because the connection is too tenuous to hold water, or because the shock effect is
not outrageous enough for the general public compared with
that of the main items.

Nicotine

Nicotine is a colourless, soluble, odourless substance with quite a
diffuse physiological effect. In small doses it stimulates activity in
the central nervous system. In larger doses it slows it down and
eventually paralyzes nerve centres. It is difficult to describe the
effect, and to determine the threshold values, because the
thresholds are different for different nerve regions. The same
doses give, for instance, one reaction in the peripheral ganglia
and another in the central nervous system.

Bodily functions are controlled by two influences: stimulus
and inhibition. Just as an arm is bent by one set of muscles and
stretched by another set, so are functions controlled. The control
occurs mainly in two ways: by hormones circulating in the blood
and through the nerves. Impulses from outside may produce
direct reactions in the tissue, as well as release them through the
brain or inferior nerve centres. A bee sting leads to swelling of
the bitten area, but, before that, there is an immediate reflex
movement of the arm. After that, there is conscious movement
via the brain, after careful consideration, which waves the arm
and causes the voice to say 'Ouch, I've been stung.'

Many stimuli are too weak by themselves to produce any
reaction, but irritation can build up, so that above a certain level
a reaction eventually occurs. The telephone ringing a couple of
times in the night may not wake you, but if the caller persists and
lets it ring twenty or thirty times you probably will wake up.
Conversely, sometimes the mechanism tires if a stimulus is re-

peated too often, and then the reaction does not occur until a certain time has passed, a resting period (the refractory period). The fatigue may be localized to the nerve as well as the organ, which may each have their special refractory period. Under such circumstances, nicotine (or some other substance) may intervene, partly stimulating, partly inhibiting, depending on the dosage.

Many functions are influenced and controlled by two opposed nerve systems, the sympathetic and the parasympathetic. These two systems have contrary effects on different functions; the sympathetic stimulates heart activity, which is inhibited by the parasympathetic. But the parasympathetic stimulates intestinal movements and certain secretions, which the sympathetic inhibits. The picture is made even more complex by the fact that each of the two systems is stimulated by certain substances in certain concentrations, but paralyzed by the same substances in larger concentrations, and that these shifts in reaction do not occur at the same concentration in different organs.

So if we want to test the effect of nicotine on the action of the heart, we may get one set of results from tests on isolated heart tissue, another on the whole heart, on heart-lung specimens, and quite another from the reaction of the heart in the whole organism. The latter seems to be the interesting observation in the debate about smoking, but simultaneously it gives results that are difficult to interpret, because heart action is influenced by so many other circumstances, each of which may even be influenced by the nicotine one way or the other. To understand this, we just have to think of the physiological influence on the heart of anger, fright, suspense, loathing, uneasiness, which increases or decreases the function. It may become even more complex because different individuals react differently at different times, depending on fitness, weariness, blood-sugar level, emotional condition, psychological power of resistance, and so on. What stimulates one person paralyzes another.

But it is fairly certain that a deadly dose of nicotine is about 20 to 50 mg taken at one time. However, nobody has ever died from taking in nicotine by smoking, because they never reach anywhere near this dosage. Our knowledge comes from people who have drunk a solution of nicotine, which for a time was used by gardeners as a pesticide. We also have descriptions of a few cases where small children have eaten cigarettes, and as little as the 1 mg or so of nicotine in the average cigarette is sufficient to cause death in a small child. The quantities absorbed from tobacco smoke are only fractions of this, and as the decomposition time for nicotine in the organism is very short, less than two hours, critical concentration in the blood will never be reached. After thirty minutes the concentration of nicotine in the brain, blood, and liver has fallen to half.

Nicotine is absorbed from the mucous membranes of the mouth, nose and throat, and goes directly into the blood. Intensive smoking may cause an acute but mild intoxication, with such symptoms as dizziness, headache, increased salivation, nausea, sweating, faintness, and even vomiting. But the symptoms usually vanish before treatment can be initiated, because of the rapid metabolism and elimination.

The concentration of nicotine in the blood decreases very rapidly, faster than it is broken down. Nicotine is deposited in different tissues, at the same time as it is metabolised and then combined with other compounds in the liver to form substances less poisonous and more easily excreted. The kidneys excrete these substances from the blood-stream almost immediately. The influence of nicotine in the 'effective field' is thus quite short, though traces can be demonstrated in various tissues up to eight hours after smoking. These concentrations are, however, of forensic interest only.

Demonstrating that nicotine is absorbed when tobacco is smoked is made easier by the fact that a decomposition product, cotinine, specific to tobacco, has a slightly longer half-life in the organism, and is relatively simple to detect. Cotinine analysis can be used to check information given at interviews about smoking habits, revealing that some people who claim to be non-smokers are probably lying, because cotinine has been found in their blood.

Some nicotine derivatives, specifically nitrosamines, have been found in laboratory tests to be carcinogenic, which means that they may lead to cancer growth. It cannot be denied that some carcinogenic nicotine decomposition products may be

Figure 7: The pharmacology of nicotine

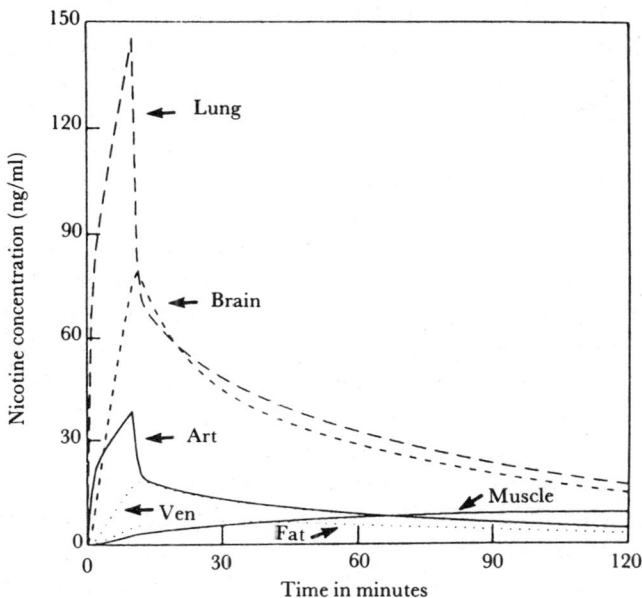

Source: Bemowitz in Rand & Thurau (eds), *The Pharmacology of Nicotine* (1987)

found after smoking, although this effect in itself has never been clinically demonstrated in humans. As so often in the tobacco debate we have to recognize that not enough is yet known on this subject to draw any definite conclusions.

A long series of studies of the psychological and physiological effects of smoking have been performed. They have shown that the psycho-physiological effect experienced after smoking one cigarette is not doubled by smoking a second cigarette, and that after this no additional effect is noticed from succeeding cigarettes. A transient acute 'immunity' has been suggested to explain why smokers limit their consumption, and why they are not driven by increasing desire for the substance because of its effect, as is the case with alcoholics and abusers of narcotics and stimulants such as 'speed'.

Carbon monoxide

Carbon monoxide is produced by any kind of burning. Stokers, nomads at their fires, employees in underground car parks, everybody gets a share of the carbon monoxide released by combustion. There are already many sources of carbon monoxide. Some can lead to acute poisoning. Tobacco provides a share of this – but it is barely significant. Carbon monoxide is odourless and is dangerous because it takes the place of oxygen in the blood: if oxygen doesn't get to the brain, you die. Normally haemoglobin becomes oxyhaemoglobin in the lungs, taking up oxygen from the air. If there is carbon monoxide in the air, it is taken up in preference to the oxygen, forming carboxyhaemoglobin. It is impossible to determine how much of the carbon monoxide found bonded to blood haemoglobin comes from a particular source. Small increases in the quantities of carboxyhaemoglobin in the blood after smoking have been measured, and this rise persists longer than nicotine levels. Higher concentrations kill by starving the brain of oxygen, as in suicide by inhaling car exhaust fumes. But the extent to which carboxyhaemoglobin is formed even during intense smoking can hardly be enough to cause headaches or drowsiness – which, by the way, are not common complaints from smokers.

Theoretically, over a longer period of time, moderate levels of carbon monoxide inhalation may result in disturbed metabolism. Fat metabolism may be affected by lower oxygenation; the penetrability of the blood capillaries may be altered; brain and heart cells may suffer; in the longer term, damage to the heart muscles may occur, as well as arteriosclerosis and stricture of the arteries.

These are the sort of effects you might expect from leaking car exhausts or old-fashioned water-heating appliances, exercising in smog, or cycling in traffic-filled city streets.

But these possibilities are offered as potentially dangerous results of tobacco smoking, although no convincing connection between these illnesses and tobacco smoking has been demonstrated.

Extensive Trials

Recently results from three comprehensive and authoritative trials have been published: the Framingham Heart Study, WHO's MONICA project, including 15 million people from 26 countries, and the Multiple Risk Factor Intervention Trials. These papers show no correlation between the distribution of the observed risk factors and heart deaths. On the contrary, the findings are paradoxical: fewer heart deaths in certain high-risk groups contradict theories about the association between the carbon monoxide burden and cardiovascular disease, in spite of what other research might have indicated. Furthermore, eliminating known risk factors in test groups (smoking, cholesterol, increased blood pressure, excess weight) resulted in hardly measurable alterations in mortality rates, and this adds to our scepticism towards the vehement campaigns against, for instance, tobacco smoking.

There have been five major studies of the effects of changing people's lifestyles, all of them comprising middle-aged males. The duration of the trials was five to twelve years. The risk factors altered by the trials were food, smoking, and blood pressure; in two of the tests, body-weight and exercise were changed as well.

After registering 828,000 man-years, the results were as follows: 1,015 deaths from heart disease in the test group, 1,049 in the control group; and 2,909 total deaths in the test group, 2,947 among the controls – a difference of 38. This means four deaths less in 10,000 man-years: that is, no practical difference.

If this is the only benefit you get from influencing people to alter their lifestyles – say, stop smoking – then it seems a bit senseless.

Constituents of tobacco smoke

The visible blue tobacco smoke consists of drops released by combustion – a so-called aerosol – most less than 1 thousandth of a millimetre in diameter, as well as some vapour and gases. This has a higher temperature than that of the room, and therefore it ascends gracefully to the ceiling, and mixes with the surrounding air.

Usually, this smoke pollution is imagined as occurring in virginal indoor air, which, however, does not exist. Firstly, indoor air is rarely purer than outdoor air, which when near traffic, in city areas, and in industrial areas, can be highly polluted by many substances. Secondly, it contains a large number of substances emanating from buildings, people, machinery, working processes, car parks, and – in private homes – from fires, stoves, oil burners, ovens, gas burners, frying pans, and electric heaters. Tobacco smoke becomes a more or less measurable contribution to this indoor air cocktail, and as a clearly visible part, with a specific odour, is easily recognizable among all the others.

The smoke aerosol carries the specific aromatic substances which are a part of the enjoyment (the taste) of tobacco smoking. Then there is the aqueous vapour and substances such as isoprene, acetaldehyde, acetone, hydrogen cyanide, toluene, acroleine, and ammonia; of no biological significance in the concentrations at which they are present in tobacco smoke. Some of the tar components of these combustion products are suspected of carcinogenicity. These substances, however, are not exclusive to tobacco smoke, and can be found from other sources. It is therefore difficult to define how large a part of them derives from which source.

The fate of the smoke in the room will be touched upon in the section about passive smoking. Many studies have been made about its effect on the smoker. Although it is claimed that the effect of nicotine – as stimulant and tranquillizer – is the actual reason for smoking, it is obvious that other factors are involved. When cigar smokers prefer to do without tobacco rather than smoke a cigarette, or smokers of one brand refuse to smoke another, even in need, it indicates that other factors exist. It is difficult to expound on these other factors because they vary so much from smoker to smoker.

Simply counting how many cigarettes someone smokes per day for how many days does not help to quantify the smoke exposure. The Banbury report describes the importance of variations in the construction of the cigarette. Rawbone refers to the importance of smoking behaviour itself. It is not enough to analyze how much there is of certain substances in the tobacco of the cigarette. Some of the substances are not released by smoking, but remain in the ashes, others are not present in the tobacco, but are formed in the combustion zone during smoking. The smoking technique itself is important, but unfortunately it is difficult to describe and even more difficult to catalogue, for instance during epidemiological studies.

During the smoking of a cigarette, substances are released from the combustion zone. The amount and combination of these are determined by the temperature in the combustion zone, and by whether you take a long, hard drag, a gentle draw, or a quick puff. It's also relevant how many puffs you can get out of each cigarette, and how much mainstream[1] smoke is exhaled by the smoker as well as how much sidestream[2] smoke is released away from the smoker by the smouldering of the cigarette itself. For this reason alone, the quantities of active substances absorbed by the smoker would be highly variable, and just as essential to establish as the number of cigarettes smoked. The smoke from the combustion zone passes through the cigarette. Immediately after the combustion zone is the distillation zone where the hot smoke stream removes volatile components – water, nicotine, etc – from the tobacco with no chemical changes. Then, further down the cigarette, the smoke is cooled down, and some of the active constituents are condensed by precipitation in the inner part of the cigarette (the condensation zone). Of importance here would be how thick the cigarette is, how firmly rolled, and not least: how much of it you smoke, since the tobacco itself serves as a filter.

If you can afford it, you might be in the habit of throwing away the stub of the cigarette before it is completely finished; some do it after having smoked only two-thirds. Others smoke

1. Mainstream smoke is produced by the smoker sucking air through the cigarette, and is given that name both before it is inhaled and after it is exhaled.
2. Sidestream smoke curls up from the combustion zone of the cigarette as it smoulders between puffs. It is produced at a lower temperature than the mainstream smoke and has some different constituents. (*Ed.*)

Figure 8:   Zones in a burning cigarette

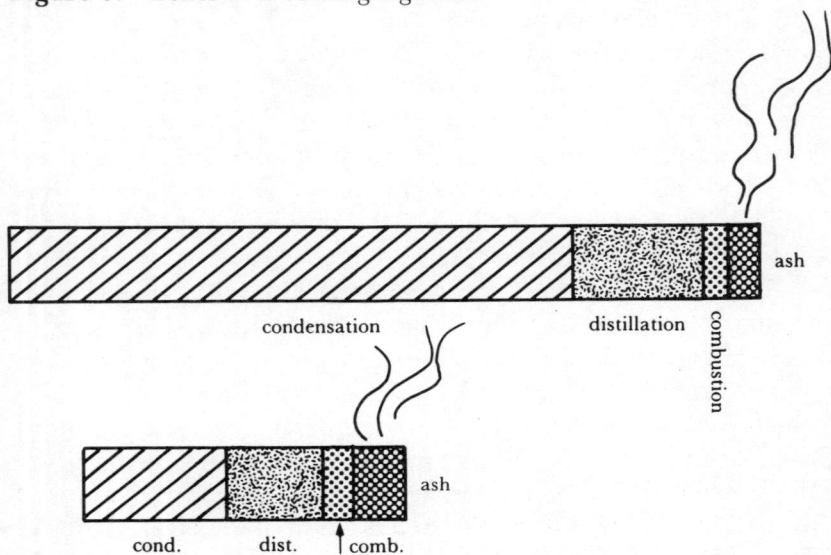

Note: when only one-third is left the condensates can be revolatilized
and thus reach the smoker

the stub right down to the filter or as closely as possible to the
end. What happens then is that part of the condensed smoke is
released again when the combustion zone reaches it. This last
part of the cigarette contains a far higher percentage and far
greater absolute quantities of the active substances than the rest
of the cigarette. The yellow nicotine-stained fingers of the pulp
novelist are not yellow from nicotine – which is colourless – but
from the tar condensate of the smoke from stubs smoked down to
the bitter end – a poor man's syndrome now rarely observed.
There is perhaps more 'poison' in three cigarettes smoked to the
last tenth than in ten smoked to a third. Such quantitative
considerations do not seem to be of much interest in the debate,
although they might be more important when evaluating the
effects of tobacco than the sheer number of smoked cigarettes.

Fairweather describes some of these variables in Wald &
Froggatt's *Nicotine, Smoking, and the Low Tar Programme*. He notes
that smoke constituents and their fate are dependent on:

(A) Cigarette construction
 Composition of the tobacco
  genetic variety
  agriculture (curing, fertilization, pesticides)
  parts of plant used
  flavouring and additives
  moisture content
 Physical design
  filtration (type of filter, ventilation)
  tobacco (density, expansion, consistency)
  cigarette (length, diameter)
  paper (porosity, additives)
(B) Individual behaviour
 Brand choice
 Brand history
 Amount smoked
  number of cigarettes per day
  number of puffs per cigarette
  puff distribution down cigarette
 Puffing behaviour
  puff volume
  puff duration
  interpuff interval
 Inhalation behaviour
  inhalation timing in relation to puff
  inhalation volume
  duration of inhalation
  normal respiratory parameters
  waste smoke
 Manner of holding cigarette
 Passive exposure
 Social/situational factors
(C) Individual physiology
 Smoking history
 Environmental interactions
 Physical status (height, weight, fitness)
 Health status (metabolic disorders, respiratory problems)
 Metabolic rates (normal or drug-induced changes)

Physical defences against toxins
Relative and variable flow-rates of biofluids
Interactions between smoke constituents and biochemicals

Smoking machines have been constructed, making possible a standardization and comparison of the released components from cigarettes. This is, however, less interesting in the face of the fact that there are so many individual ways to smoke, which makes a comparison between various smokers' exposure to different substances very difficult. It is far from sufficient to classify smokers according to the number of cigarettes per day. This would tell us less about the quantity and combination of the active compounds than those other circumstances.

8

Why do People Smoke?

This question has been examined by various scientific disciplines and on different levels – some frivolous, some serious. The literature is impressive, but my heretical common sense is pleased to note that the best answer yet produced is exactly the one it would have given: people smoke because they like it.

Apart from this excellent statement, a number of particular effects have been documented, each of which may be an argument for smoking tobacco. Electro-physiological, psycho-social, hereditary, neuro-chemical, and many other specialties have delved deeply into the problem and found explanations of why people smoke.

Instinctively, you might think that the group with the greatest interest in determining why people smoke would be advertising people in the tobacco business. But as it has been shown that advertisements don't make people start or continue smoking, and that the campaigns of the industry are only about winning shares of the existing market for some brands instead of others, the role of advertising must take a back-seat in this connection.

Psychologists and educationists would have a natural interest in the motives for smoking. Freudians would be able to say something about fixation in the oral phase, and mean that those who smoke have been weaned too soon by an unloving mother and seek compensation here. There might be a case of sexual repression, making smoking a substitute for kissing. If you cannot suck on Marilyn Monroe's lips, you can light up a Partagas – and suck on that. . . .

But what pressures encourage beginners and who teaches them to smoke? Group behaviour and peer pressure have been examined, as has identification with hero figures or father figures. Weak egos, it is claimed, seek strength and security in smoking, copying national figures or idols of the media world.

Sociologists note influences from cultural levels and regional traditions, social environment, profession, and family, and see smoking as a distinct social-dependent behaviour pattern. Something like this is confirmed by the distribution of smokers and non-smokers by gender and social strata, jobs and acquaintances. Psychology recedes in favour of sociology when it is noted that low-status groups and townspeople smoke more, mostly cigarettes; that career and media people smoke cigarettes to a greater extent than others (heavy smokers); that the pipe is generally preferred in certain circles, and that the cigar has a rather local social distribution, apart from Latin America where the cigar was born and is widely smoked.

There is also the experience that apparently well-entrenched smoking habits can change when a person's life situation is drastically changed: for instance, on marriage to a non-smoker, on moving into a job in a non-smoking environment, or upon religious conversion.

Powerful lobbies are involved in getting smokers to abandon their vice; health protagonists motivate their activity with the conviction that tobacco is harmful, seeking selective proof wherever they can. This includes attempts at prevention from well-intentioned medical people as well as conversion attempts by missionaries. As for the smokers at whom these efforts are directed, they cope for as long as possible with their irritation over these efforts to make them do something they do not want to do. The majority of smokers still try to ignore all these attacks. They want to be left in peace.

There are many models of smoking behaviour – Eysenck's diathesis-stress model, Tomkin's affect-control model, for example. Familial smoking patterns are offered as predisposing factors, and so are personality structures, emotional bases, situational motives; smoking has been explained as learnt through classical teaching, or by imitation mechanisms, socio-psychological influences in youth, and as a means to gain contact or social acceptance.

There have been many studies and reports without any motive showing up as convincingly central. There is probably something in all of it; elements are more significant for some people than for others. An interesting observation: very few people get pleasure from smoking in darkness; apparently they need to see the smoke. This might indicate the totality of the whole smoking situation: the cosiness of the ritual, the sight, the smell, the company, the meditation. This aspect has surprised me, for one, who would not have attached any immediate importance to the sight of the smoke.

Of the more concrete studies about smokers' motives, we can refer to the report from the International Symposium on Electrophysiological Effects of Nicotine in Paris 1978, to Ney & Gales's anthology about *Smoking and Human Behaviour*, to the many papers from all over the world demonstrating various effects of nicotine: improved learning, level of accomplishment, and attention; anxiety mitigation and relaxation; and positive influences registered by electro-encephalograms, energy conversion, and so on.

Somewhat less specialized reviews of the whole problem are found in, for instance, *Smoking and Society*, edited by Tollison, or in Wetterer & v. Troschke's *Smoker Motivation*, but apart from these there are other earnest researchers, whose names recur through the years, and who add to the puzzle bit by bit (as Warburton says: *The Puzzle of Nicotine Use*).

I myself do not feel dependent upon smoking. My consumption is constant from year to year. I consider it a pleasant quality of my daily life, which I choose despite all allegations about health risks. (By the way, I am seventy-two years of age and in excellent health, and therefore I do not care very much). But I am disturbed by smoking restrictions which seem to hit me in exactly those situations when you need a smoke: waiting for people, trains or planes, riding the latter, or otherwise passive outside the daily routine. What are you supposed to do – pick your nose, read idiotic magazines? You cannot do anything serious in a waiting room, in a phase of life which is a vacuum: when what you want to do is light a good cigar and feel that life is not just going down the drain. . . . It is in exactly these situations that you face prohibitions and restrictions, and it is exactly then you feel where some of your motivation for smoking may come from.

The controversy has taken a new direction in recent years: featuring nicotine as an addictive substance, even comparable with heroin and cocaine. The protagonist of this standpoint has been the main inspiration of the fight against tobacco, the former US Surgeon General. The argument is not so much about the actual effects of tobacco smoking as it is about making tobacco fit into the definition of addictive substances. The US Surgeon General asserts that tobacco is addictive and then formulates a definition of addiction which embraces tobacco. That it does not fit the other known narcotic substances, and moreover seems meaningless, does not stop it from turning up in the debate with great weight. The same technique is applied by the Royal Society of Canada which simply advocates a novel definition of 'addiction'. The American Psychiatric Association follows suit, producing a list of diagnostic criteria to help recognize withdrawal symptoms in smokers who stop smoking.

Those of us who work with drug abuse and drug addiction have developed a number of quite simple and easily describable criteria of addiction. It would be reasonable, one should think, to examine whether a substance fits into the existing definition; not to alter the definition so that it fits a certain substance.

A person's relationship with any substance, be it food, drink or drug, is based primarily on the wish to have it. A psychological dependence may arise, so you get used to the substance and miss it if you must do without. It may be a spice for your food, or peppermint, or honey on your morning rolls. This dependence is, however, not so deep that it will influence your work, and the lack of the substance at times will not influence your usual level of performance. You may get irritated about it, it may bother you. But you function normally.

When psychologically dependent, habituated, you always have freedom of choice in relation to the substance; you may choose whether you want to take the trouble of going out for a pack of cigarettes, you may refrain from it if it is too long a journey or it is raining.

It is quite different if there is physical dependence. Then you have no choice. You need the substance to function, like a thirsty person needs water. And you function badly, or not at all, if you do not get your needs satisfied. You simply get sick if you do not get it.

Your organism has not only accepted the alien substance, it has made it a part of its metabolism, and will react if the substance is suddenly not there. It is a characteristic mechanism of addiction that the organism accepts the alien substance, and that it stops reacting defensively against it. Another typical mechanism, specific to addiction, is based on this: increased tolerance. There is no reaction to larger and larger doses of the substance, indeed still larger doses are necessary to obtain the same effect as was obtained by smaller doses previously. (I once had a morphine-abusing patient in a Copenhagen prison who tolerated ten times the lethal doses without any other effect than getting 'high' from it.)

Those who have reached high tolerance levels and are addicted to large doses of the substance, get sick when they are suddenly deprived of it. For each substance, typical symptoms of withdrawal are described which are different for, say, alcohol, morphine, or amphetamine.

The seriously humiliating withdrawal symptoms are both physical (sweating, dizziness, palpitation, shivering, vomiting) and psychological (anxiety, hallucinations, delusions, confusion, psychotic conditions). It is the fear of these reactions that drives the addict to try and procure the substance at any price. The physical demand to maintain 'normality' results in an intense desire for the substance, called 'craving'.

Craving eventually results in the normally law-abiding breaking laws to finance their addiction: burglary, theft, hold-ups, fraud, and embezzlement. This moral shift is often accompanied by character changes and mental dissolution, with financial collapse and social deprivation.

It is a common misconception that this sequence is caused by the particular substances. But they have no diabolical power in themselves. Most people who consume alcohol do not become addicted. Many patients are doped with potent drugs for therapeutic purposes (treatment of post-operative pain, for instance) without becoming drug addicts. The addiction is a function of the reactions of certain people to specific situations, perhaps a latent crisis in a personal situation more significant than the chemistry of the substance.

So we can list the respective criteria and place tobacco and alcohol or drugs against them. The picture will be like this:

Table 3: Criteria for distinguishing between habituation and addiction

	Habituation	Addiction
Want	+	+
Freedom of choice	+	−
Psychological dependence	+	+
Physical dependence	−	+
increased tolerance	−	+
escalation of dosage	−	+
withdrawal	−	+
craving	−	+
Moral deterioration	−	+
Intellectual reduction	−	+
Mental dissolution	−	+
Social collapse	−	+

Tobacco consumption fits the 'habituation' side much better than the 'addiction' side. The difference is obvious between smoking and drug abuse exemplified by alcoholics and morphine addicts. The fact that most smokers smoke the same quantities year after year suggests that nicotine is not addictive. You don't get people increasing the dose. Its duration in the blood is less than an hour, but smokers (even heavy smokers) do not wake up every hour during the night with withdrawal symptoms, craving for a smoke. Finally, giving up smoking is not usually helped by nicotine-containing preparations. Nicotine chewing-gum to help you give up smoking is probably less important than your will. It may be that chewing gum *per se* (with no pharmacological content) may substitute for the habit of using the mouth.

Comparing tobacco to, say, cocaine is therefore directly misleading, and can only be based on an ignorance of these matters – or is it a cynical deception when such serious and false arguments have to be produced to discourage the use of tobacco?

9

A Frivolous Essay about Smokers and Non-Smokers

'*Laus Tabacci*', the classic praise of all the virtues of tobacco, is pure poetry. It does not talk about lungs, but speaks directly to the heart. It is a declaration of love, and even the most inveterate anti-smokers must allow us the right to love the fragrant herb and its gentle blue smoke.

We have luxuriated in it at the lakeside, holding a fishing rod; relaxed with it over a mug of coffee by the log-fire, where it kept gnats at bay; survived with it as we lay hove-to cowering on the locker seat in a dank cabin while gales raged around the boat; waited with it for restless hours outside the maternity ward; pondered lofty topics with it among good friends reclining in deep armchairs. And we have died with it, like my old father at the age of ninety-three; when nothing else was to his taste, he enjoyed his last cigar, and declared philosophically that were he offered another year of life if he stopped smoking, he would decline.

We have been happy with tobacco and would have been very reluctant to do without it. It has added to the quality of life in this vale of tears, and has reconciled us to that life when it was sour. It has sweetened life when it was good. And we have enjoyed it.

Fanatics

The anti-smokers are fanatics. They lead a crusade based on belief. They have to overplay their cards so they can cover their rears in their aggressive assaults. They disregard the need for proof; their arguments are allegations, and they stick rigidly to their views, despite any facts to the contrary. Their indifference to the evidence gives them unlimited scope for allegations of all kinds, and makes counter-argument seem cumbersome and stupid. How can you prove that pixies do not exist . . .?

This makes debate hopeless, and ensures that publications like this and other books don't join the fray. But, at least, I hope they will lend moral support to those bombarded by propaganda, to those defenceless tobacco lovers, intimidated and threatened into changing the habits and pleasures of a lifetime.

One can only guess what their motives are. It seems most likely that they simply hate smokers (or one smoker?). One of their arguments is that they are working for our own best interest – to prevent our downfall. But when we observe their activities, is it so convincing that they love us so much that they would sacrifice so much to save us, against our will and despite our protests? We have not asked them for their care, and do not believe in the necessity of it – on the contrary, we have asked not to have any of it. Why do they, then, keep on butting in on us, bothering us?

Classification

I have often wondered whether it might be possible to determine what makes a smoker or a non-smoker. Many columns of newsprint, and many books (see References pp. 135ff.) have been devoted to the question: why do people smoke? Half of the answer may be found in this question: why do some people not smoke. . . ?

Might it not be reasonable to make a clear distinction between non-smokers – people who don't smoke from sensible motives, and don't care if others do – and anti-smokers, the belligerent enemies of tobacco, the missionaries, the crusaders? At those confrontations which are now so popular with the media, I have often been offered the general observation that smokers seem so cheerful, tolerant, and domestic, while anti-smokers are fierce, aggressive, and surly. Even I have been told that, at my ad-

vanced age and after a long career as a smoker, I am evidently
healthier and more agile than my anaemic, strained, and
shrivelled opponents. And, of course, I find that amusing.

Many studies have been made of the distribution of smokers
and non-smokers: men/women, town/country, blue collar/white
collar, educated/non-educated, high status/low status, pyknics/
asthenics, and so on. Apart from some rough sociological and
geographical differences, these studies have come to no definite
conclusions. The relaxed, recumbent smoker having either
solved his problems or letting them rest unsolved for a while, is
both a literary platitude and straight reality. From the viewpoint
of mental hygiene, this seems a reasonable and therefore healthy
reaction.

But the problem solver contemplating his task is also typically
a smoker. A great scientist like Niels Bohr can support his
wandering through the labyrinths of knowledge by holding on to
a fixed point: his pipe. It is true that many take to tobacco in
stressful and worrying situations. These are, I think, harassed
persons resorting to the symbol of peace and equilibrium, remi-
niscing on pleasant moments beyond the immediate problems.

The cowboys in Marlboro Country smoke cigarettes, but they
are advertisement cowboys. 'Real' cowboys – we know from
John Wayne and colleagues – smoke cigarillos. But how they are
able to draw long weeds from their breast pockets after a long
day's ride and light up without problems is a puzzle to me. Mine
would be broken if I treated them like that. There's a little fiction
in that, I suspect. Cowboys, other than the clean and newly
shaved in advertisements and motion pictures, would roll their
cigarettes themselves, I am sure, even from fluff and tobacco
scraps – in whatever paper is at hand. The thin paper from the
Old Testament was very popular with us during the war. Cowboys may be too pious to dare use the Scriptures or the Psalm
Book in such a sacrilegious way . . .

Could Al Capone have achieved and kept his American
empire together without fat cigars? Majestic, authoritative and
stately are attributes associated with the cigar (which is never
smoked down to a stub). Jean Gabin with a cigar – no, Caporal,
and typically it had to be a Caporal. And Humphrey Bogart?

Well, what else than Virginia. Marlene Dietrich? I have never wanted to be a cigarette so much as when she languidly toys with one (usually Turkish) – when she really plays the role, even with a long holder, but there I quit. I would never be that cigarette – and if I were something else, I would not have the slightest notion what I should talk to such a lady about.

There is plenty of scope here for the anthropologist and the taxonomist, and more psychology than perhaps one suspects. The way people smoke is an expression of their character: many people gesticulate more clearly with a cigarette; veil themselves in the smoke from the cigar; are attached to their pipe. They love it, it is part of their persona, marked by their teeth, worn by their hands.

The smoker becomes a picture of submission. He is reclining, his hands are open and safely engaged in peaceful pursuits. No attacks are expected of him. Is it possible to imagine Hitler smoking? Could he be imagined just as insane and aggressive if he had been able to lean back with his feet on his desk and a cigar in his mouth? These SS types looking like Himmler's twins with their stare, their rigid posture, their tight lips, could they be imagined as so evil and so stupid if they had been pipe smokers? On the other hand, the Junker officers of the Wehrmacht could juggle with a cigarette and its smoke with the elegance of a man of the world from the turn of the century – another kind of human being.

It is possible that Stalin was just as insane and despotic as any of them, but, at any rate, with his pipe he was able to live up to a human image of a certain joviality and convivality. The pipe revealed another ideal: good old Uncle Joe – and in this alone there is a significant difference. The Nazis wanted to be terrifying, ruthless, and went to great lengths to look like that. Therefore never tobacco, relaxation, peacefulness. No pipe, never a cigar. The fear of becoming dependent on such people was justified.

Would Fidel Castro have succeeded in his revolution without big cigars? you may wonder. An army of bearded men with big cigars in their mouths behind the sights of a gun are difficult to cope with. This is obvious to everybody, friend and enemy.

There is propaganda value in the cigar. Maybe Churchill didn't really like cigars, but being an old fox he might have seen it as an excellent way to convince people of his resolve and faith that everything would turn out all right, despite blitz and blockade and defeat.

There are thousands of lonely old people living in miserable conditions, without hope and with very little contact with the outside world. Many of these will tell you that without their cup of coffee and a smoke, their lives would be unbearable. To make people dislike this harmless benefit of life seems not only senseless – but evil. Burdening this pathetic prop with negative values and blaming it for the minor and major ailments of age seems foolish, quite apart from being unproven and improbable. Tobacco smoking has an inestimable social value that should be respected and appreciated. The suicide rate for Danish men over the age of sixty-five is already twice as high as the average for the population as a whole. Is that what we want . . .?

Has anybody ever in real life or in the literature been seen crying with a cigar in his mouth? As long as you smoke, you are invincible. A cigar is an expression of surplus, wealth, balance, of being in control. And cigars are like smiles – a certain mood is normally believed to be expressed by them. But do not underestimate the opposite effect. Forcing a smile may actually make you feel better; smoking a cigar can stimulate extra resources.

Democratic debate?

Debate is part of our culture. Debate teaches its participants to listen – to try and understand. They also learn to express their opinions and attitudes in words that can be understood by others. Not least do they learn that for words to be worth listening to, they must be based on knowledge, on reality. Debate is a cornerstone of the democratic process. Until the pros and cons have been elucidated and expressed we cannot come to competent conclusions. And as for confidence in democracy, it is necessary for the consequences of newly acquired knowledge to be taken to their logical conclusion. Our confidence in Norway's parliament, for example, would be stimulated if it turned out, in a few years' time, that the morbidity and death rate had not changed with their restrictive legislation against tobacco, and if then they repealed the legislation. It would be even better if new attempts were made to legislate against the *real* pollutors.

Respecting, as we do, the democratic process, we listen to the anti-smokers. But as their arguments are often distorted, their 'facts' tendentious, and their conclusions illogical or improbable, we consider them unreliable. And because they are not receptive to arguments (if they listen to them at all), we are unlikely to be on speaking terms with them.

This is all within their human rights – as we have the right to refuse them. It is not until they want to force us, through legislation, to their views, that we have to protest and seek to stop them.

10

The Harmful Effects of Passive Smoking

No permanent effects have ever been demonstrated. It is true that passive smoking may cause smarting eyes, irritation of the nose and throat, headache, and may have an annoying smell — but these are matters of subjective inconvenience. What annoys some people, leaves others unaffected; all we are left with are people's *claims* about degrees of inconvenience. And these change according to the situation and the attitude of the person asking the questions.

It could be maintained (although it seems a bit unlikely) that passive smoking caused backache, which would make it painful and intolerable to be with smokers, and that this would motivate prohibition of smoking. Nobody is able to measure pain in the back.[1] The pain-meter has never been invented. Backache as well as general inconvenience in connection with passive smoking are assertions that one can take note of or remain sceptical towards. The degree of effect cannot be demonstrated.

We must be considerate of each other. The question is how to weigh consideration. We know the problem in practice, for instance, with asthmatics whose condition is influenced by dust, carpeting, wall coverings, plants, and pets. How much money are we to spend on altering buildings in order to spare these patients their attacks? How much are we supposed to change the world so that they, too, can live in it, and function reasonably? When are they to be declared so handicapped that they cannot be accepted as normal and live among other people . . . that they

1. In early 1992 a US machine was used in a British court for the first time to give an objective assessment of the extent of physical injury to the back in a claim for damages. (*Ed.*)

'must live with' their handicap? There is no definite solution to such questions. They must be under constant debate. And we must realize that the human considerations we would like to show are constantly limited by economic possibilities.

Non-smoking spouses

In 1981 the debate changed radically because a novel factor was brought in. Hirayama reported that non-smoking Japanese women married to smoking men got lung cancer more frequently than women married to non-smoking men. This introduced a new and moral factor to the controversy. Smokers bring to their families and social relations the risk of contracting deadly diseases! The very same year, this finding was confirmed by the studies of Trichopoulos who found similar tendencies in a Greek group. These reports, immediately and with authority, were included in the US Surgeon General's reports, which are taken as gospel by the authorities and anti-smoking publicists in many countries.

That same year, interestingly enough, Garfinkel (American Cancer Society) published a report covering 180,000 American women, in which he found that lung cancer mortality among non-smoking women with smoking spouses compared to those with non-smoking spouses showed that there were no statistically significant differences. Neither this nor several later studies with similar results, nor extensive critical revisions, have been referred to in the press, nor have they influenced the US Surgeon General's crusade, nor have they had any impact on the debate whatsoever, apart from the one in scientific circles.

Hirayama (at Japan's National Cancer Centre Research Institute) based his examination upon interviews with 265,118 adults from 29 districts over a period of fourteen years, from 1966 to 1979. There was a 90 per cent response to the questionnaires, which dealt with many subjects, including food and diseases. Hirayama found that 72 per cent of all couples gave information about the smoking habits of both spouses. Out of 91,540 married women, he found that 245 died from lung cancer, 174 of whom

(71 per cent) were non-smokers. These 174 deaths were then related to the smoking habits of their spouses, and he found a majority of these women were married to smokers.

Hirayama's research has become a favourite example among professionals of unreliable documentation, of bad science, of overinterpretation of defective data. Hirayama has never verified the diagnoses at death; the returns of the questionnaires have never been controlled or followed up; there is no verification or quantification of the smoking habits of the spouses; the observed group was recruited from the most strongly industrialized area in Japan and was not representative of the general population. The control group is not comparable, because there is an unusual proportion of elderly women. The statistical treatment of the material is full of errors, and the prognosis on the basis of findings is incorrect. Finally, apart from these evident biases, no correction has been made for complicating factors, such as housing conditions, cooking facilities, heating, duration of partnership, and so on.

When fifty scientists and physicians gathered for a meeting in Vienna in 1984 to discuss the evidence that passive smoking may cause lung cancer, everybody – with one exception – agreed that no proof existed of any connection. The exception was Dr Takesi Hirayama.

Hirayama's allegations are based on these women reporting, after having been asked once, that they do not smoke and that their spouses do smoke, and this has never been checked. Nothing about previous circumstances, nothing about the duration of their spouses' smoking or the length of the partnership, nothing that tells us how much was smoked, for how long, and where. The diagnosis of lung cancer is hearsay and unverified. At boring scientific conferences a favourite way of cheering up the audience was to submit a new critique of the Hirayama study, as Ahlborn and Überla did in London in 1988. To everybody's vast amusement, they showed that even if one accepted all the errors and uncertainties of Hirayama's data, and overlooked all the biases, a correct statistical treatment of the material could lead to the opposite conclusion.

As for the Trichopoulos study, it is not taken seriously – and

Trichopoulos himself has reservations about it, if for no other reason than that the material is too small for any conclusion to be drawn. There were 77 non-smokers compared to 225 controls, without verification of diagnosis, and procured by one and the same interviewer in interviews that were neither blind nor double-blind. A paradoxical result was that the incidence of cancer cases among interviewees exposed to their spouse's smoke were greatest at low consumption rates, decreasing among heavy smoking spouses (comparing evaluations of one-digit figures!).

Garfinkel himself dared not draw any conclusions from his large study. He found none of the differences were of statistical significance, and concluded that non-smokers married to smokers showed very little if any increased risk of lung cancer. The presumed 'relative risk' was 1.4 for non-smoking partners of men who smoked less than 20 cigarettes a day, while decreasing to 1.0 when they smoked more than that. Garfinkel said: 'Passive smoking is a political issue, but hardly a reasonable measure for health policy.'

Garfinkel published data on 134 cases of lung cancer among non-smokers interviewed on admission to hospital. Of these, 92 had been exposed to spousal smoking, 42 not exposed to spousal smoking. The conclusion may be obvious – until one realizes that 134 flat-footed subjects would show the same distribution, with a clear majority exposed to spousal smoking, since this is a normal distribution figure for the population as a whole. Almost parallel results were found by Garfinkel in his control group of 402 non-smokers who had not got lung cancer: 266 with a smoking spouse, 136 with a non-smoking spouse.

But only almost. The distribution 92/42 is a bit larger than 266/136, namely a ratio of 1 to 1.12 ('relative odds'). This shows with statistical significance that there is a greater risk of lung cancer among non-smokers if they have a smoking spouse – assuming the figures procured by interviews are reliable.

We know that various interviewers get different results. We also know that the same persons may answer differently at various points in time. For instance, pronounced differences have been noted in the answers to questions about smoking habits among relatives of people who have died from lung cancer.

Answers from surviving spouses show equal numbers among these of smokers and non-smokers, which means that no influence from spouses' smoking has been found. But other relatives, typically children, give quite another description of the smoking habits of the spouse of the deceased, giving three times as many smokers as non-smokers in the same subjects, showing a considerably increased risk from a smoking spouse – plus a moral burden on the 'guilty' person.

I once did a survey by anonymous questionnaire among fifteen-year-old schoolgirls about the time they started having sex. About 50 per cent reported having started before the age of fifteen. Questioning the same girls two years later gave a median age for sexual début as seventeen.

A woman admitted to the lung department for observation reported that she had no smoking spouse. Her partner could, however, at his daily visits hardly bear not being able to smoke in the ward and had to go out on to the staircase once or twice during each visit. When told this, the woman explained: 'Well, yes, but we are not married.'

So much for the reliability of studies using interviews.

Table 4: A small hypothetical shift . . . if only 4 per cent of the people in the Garfinkel study were lying the figures in brackets could be the actual values.

	Lung cancer	No lung cancer
	134	402
Passive smoking	92 (87)	266
No passive smoking	42 (47)	136
Relative odds: 1.12 (0.94)		

Source: Schneider (1990)

If we suppose that in Garfinkel's material only as many as 5 out of 134 gave a false answer – whether they misunderstood the question or simply lied (remember, we are in a lung department and the question may be: You don't smoke tobacco, do you?) – then we get 87 having been exposed to passive smoking and 47 who have not, out of the 134 cases of lung cancer. Relative odds would then be 0.94 – statistically significant, showing that there is a decreased risk for non-smokers married to smokers (Table 4).

The example tells us nothing about the risk of contracting lung cancer from passive smoking, but it does show how easy it is to draw false conclusions from the data of badly designed studies.

This phenomenon has repeated itself over and over again. New life was brought to the debate when in 1980 White & Froeb measured the lung function of smokers and non-smokers and found that non-smokers exposed to tobacco smoke at work for twenty years had reduced lung function, a result that the US Surgeon General adopted and broadcast to all authorities and specialists.

That White and Froeb were criticized and immediately re-pudiated in professional circles made very little impression (Adlkofer, Huber, Friedman, Aviado). The researchers had used carbon monoxide as the index for smoke influence, although this is not characteristic of tobacco smoke but of innumerable other sources. They had not made corrections for the carbon monoxide content of the air at the observed localities without a mix of tobacco smoke, nor had they gathered a proper control group. Moreover, the results were apparently only applicable after 3,000 cases had been excluded from the study, for unstated reasons. At the same time, a series of analogous studies from all over the world found that no connection could be found.

In parallel with this has been the argument over the effects of passive smoking on the heart. Aronow published, as the result of his research, proof that angina pectoris pains presented them-selves at an earlier and more severe stage among patients who had been exposed to tobacco smoke. His material was 10 angina pectoris patients. Despite professional criticism, Aronow's re-sults have been referred to as facts in the US Surgeon General's reports from 1979, 1980, and 1981. Characteristic of this course of events is that although Aronow's study was shown to be based on falsified data (Benignus *et al.*) weighty arguments based on Aronow's results continued to appear in the debate.

Apart from scepticism justified by experience, in connection with the reliability of studies based on interviews, we know of simple biases and erroneous classifications that constantly

appear, making conclusions from the material dubious and useless. Let us take such a simple matter as distributing the patient
base between smokers and non-smokers. We have previously
pointed to the problem of simply defining the concept. But even
after a crystal-clear definition, it turns out to be impossible to
avoid erroneous classification. Many people who report being
non-smokers (for moral reasons in relation to treatment) have
turned out to have such a high level of blood cotinine that it can
only have come from active smoking; so these cases are wrongly
classified. Furthermore, 40 per cent of women classified as non-
smokers have actually smoked in periods of their lives. And,
according to Garfinkel, many who get 'tobacco-related' diseases
have a tendency to deny smoking – more frequently than controls with diseases never associated with smoking. On top of this,
Friedman *et al.* found that 47 per cent of non-smoking women
married to smokers had never been exposed to passive smoking
at all; while 40 per cent of non-smoking women married to
non-smokers reported having been exposed to passive smoking
outside their homes. The value of the parameter 'smoking
spouse' has thus been demonstrated as an actual mis-classi-
fication. And where then should all the accusatory material end
up . . .?

Lee *et al.* show in an extensive survey the dependence upon
method. In interviews with 12,693 patients, they tried to quantify and specify exposure to tobacco smoke, which is what
Hirayama and Trichopoulos and others have failed to do. They
recorded when the marriage or partnership had begun, if (and
when) it ended, number of units (cigarettes, cigars, pipes)
smoked by the partner during the previous twelve months,
estimated maximum time for this, second and succeeding mar-
riages, estimation of latent intervals between exposure and
disease, quantification of smoking according to a four-point scale
(much, normal, little, not at all) and influence by other sources –
work, transportation, leisure time, for example. It is self-evident
that an increasing number of questions and increasing
differentiation will cause increasing uncertainty of responses,
and comparisons will be increasingly unclear. At the same time,
the test material, differentiated into respective groups, becomes

smaller, too, and thus the statistical computations unreliable. Lee *et al.* came to the conclusion that the relative risk of developing lung cancer in relation to smoking of spouse was 0.80. Which means that non-smokers married to smokers were 20 per cent less exposed to this risk than non-smokers married to non-smokers – quite a confusing result!

As late as November 1988 a major WHO review of everything then published about passive smoking concluded that, until then, there were not sufficient studies (there were at the time more than 1,000) to prove a connection between passive smoking and lung cancer.

Such things – negative findings, doubts, and contradictory criteria – do not penetrate very far into the public consciousness because they are never mentioned by the protagonists in the debate. Which cannot, for that reason, be taken seriously.

Ping . . . pong . . .

The whole tobacco debate looks like a game of ping-pong where the serve constantly comes from the anti-smokers. One study shows how harmful smoking and passive smoking are, the next one shows that the first one is not tenable – ping, pong.

So it goes, time after time. The anti-smokers offer a proof. To rebut it there are those who want to defend the method and reliability of their science: scientists, not pro-smokers. Nobody wants to (and nobody can) prove that tobacco smoking is harmless. But many feel obliged to repudiate trivial or futile studies maintaining that it is harmful. And so it goes . . . ping, pong. . . .

It also seems as if those involved divide into two groups: among the anti-smokers there are some who start out from the conviction that there is a real risk, and see it as their task to demonstrate and prove this by all means. The other front consists of scientists dominated by doubt who realize that they know nothing and therefore want to be guided by their science. It is precisely their feelings of doubt that make them check their opponents' cocksure statements. Can it be correct that . . .?

In science there should never be – but it cannot be denied that there often are – differences between planning and carrying out a project to demonstrate there *is* a connection, and doing the study to see *if* there's a connection. This difference often seems critical to the results of the study.

And even to the layman it is obvious that the debate is plagued with subjectivity. Prognoses from unproved figures – ping. Over-interpretation of test results – ping. Wrong technique, false method, distortion of multifactorial priorities, generalization on limited observations – ping. Erroneous statistical treatment, careless prognoses – ping. You claim to show something about tobacco smoking and risks – we maintain that nobody knows enough to say what you are saying – pong. Ping-pong.

It is, however, on the basis of this insufficient knowledge that the public at large chooses sides, that good people and school children are brainwashed, that sentiments are worked up, cat-egorical positions become set in stone, emotions mobilized. And it is on this basis that we are given statutes and statutory instruments that penetrate deeply into working life, patterns of behaviour and social conditions, and limit citizens' freedom to choose for themselves.

As for the few smokers' associations, they are definitely on the defensive. None of them seeks to persuade others to smoke. They seek only to defend their right to make their own choices – without officious interference from over-enthusiastic tutors.

11
Indoor Air

When somebody wants to document the impact of smoking on indoor air, it seems that he simply has to compare smoke-filled air with smoke-free air. In order to do this, he needs to make one or several measurements to make such comparisons possible. The entire examination of the problem becomes extremely technical, a long series of experiments and considerations about measurement equipment and methods, about analyses and variables, and later on a discussion of the validity of it all and of its possible influence upon human well-being and health under such conditions.

This part of the problem is dominated by technicians, building engineers, chemists, architects, ventilation experts, bioanalysts, inventors of equipment and measurements. One of the difficulties is not only to find a national language in which the participants may communicate with little restraint (English is generally chosen), but also to find a technical language in which all these different specialties can convey their very special professional experience. Physicians, chemists, electrotechnicians, mathematicians, engineers: how far can they understand each other's professional problems, treatments, and results? Some misconceptions and misinterpretations come from this problem, and make demands on understanding and good will. Where it is difficult to make anybody understand, it is nearly impossible to prevent somebody from misunderstanding – especially if they actually want to do so.

Many of the considerations about the health impacts of passive smoking rest upon algebraic reckoning. If the air in a room contains tobacco smoke corresponding to the smoke from X number of cigarettes, the harmful effect must be equal to this. Here it is presupposed that the damaging effect of smoking X number of cigarettes is well documented (which it is not), and that we can reliably measure non-smokers' exposure to tobacco smoke, and can compare it to the smoking of cigarettes – which is also not possible.

Finally, it is assumed that substances found in indoor air in a room where tobacco is smoked are the same that are inhaled through smoking – which is not at all the case.

You can try to elucidate the problem by chemical analyses of the air, taking into account how much this measurement is influenced by factors such as the size of the room, ventilation, humidity, temperature, decomposition of respective substances, adsorption of particles and gases on surfaces (persons, furniture, walls, curtains), absorption of gases and vapour. If comparisons are to be made – or results to be transferred to normal situations – selected standard rooms with variable conditions are needed. But there will still be a considerable uncertainty in comparing such results from experiments to daily-life reality, with its extremely changeable conditions, to which a non-smoker is exposed during periods of his life that may be decisive for the development of diseases.

The substances inhaled by a smoker through the cigarette (cigar, pipe), 'mainstream smoke', are different from the ones released into the air by the smouldering of the cigarette ('sidestream smoke'). This latter smoke is released at low temperature in the combustion zone and is not filtered through the cigarette. It therefore contains another combination of the same substances as mainstream smoke – some of them in higher concentrations even.

ETS (Environmental Tobacco Smoke) is a measure of the tobacco smoke in the air of a room, and is what passive smokers are exposed to. ETS is a mixture of sidestream smoke and exhaled smoke released by the smoker after 'using' the smoke. ETS depends upon the intensity of smoking. It is evident that the same amount of smoke in one room would give half the first ETS level in a room twice as large. It is also evident that ETS depends on the renewal of air, the ventilation, and on the size and number of absorbing surfaces, persons, pieces of furniture, and so on, in the room.

The widely different and contradictory estimates of the contribution of a fixed number of cigarettes to the ETS in a room, are due to the fact that estimates are made from different starting points. An estimate that staying in a smoke-filled room (a pub, a billiard room) for a certain time would correspond to smoking so many cigarettes, is therefore just as arbitrary as the calculation that passive smoking exposes a person to two thousandths as much substance as actively smoking X number of cigarettes – merely because under certain chosen conditions the concentration of substances in ETS is 1/2000 of that in mainstream smoke.

ETS is dependent on room size, the number of cigarettes smoked, and ventilation. It might therefore be maintained that the problem of ETS is simply a question of sufficient ventilation. And considering how many other undetected substances contribute to the pollution of indoor air, it could be statutorily ordered that, as an indicator of proper ventilation, tobacco must be smoked in every public office and at every working place. If the smoke became a nuisance, this would be an expression of insufficient ventilation!

Measuring the cotinine content of the blood of passive smokers and comparing it with that of smokers would probably give the most reliable estimate of the possible health risk, to which the former are exposed. The various parameters – maxima, mean values, thresholds, and time intervals – still give ample latitude for estimates and interpretations. Would two-thousandths of the smoke exposure mean a two-thousandths' risk of the appropriate disease, and how would this work in a physiological sense in relation to a series of other influences?

We are here faced with the problem of demonstrating an increase in risk of two-thousandths. On top of this, there is the question: who would be bothered to determine this – considering all the other risk factors of modern existence.

Sick buildings

To prove causal connection, the observed persons must not have been affected by other factors that may be responsible for the development of their condition, and which could confuse the issue. As this is all about exposure over a number of years, it is virtually impossible to set up such circumstances.

With the present increasing consciousness about environmental issues, there also arises an increasing understanding of the importance of indoor air in which modern man spends such a large part of his existence. From this comes a powerful interest in analyses and assessment of indoor air, and in finding out what this means for our well-being and health. The understanding of risks from open sewers, polluted drinking water, and vermin has now been enlarged to encompass ventilation, synthetic building materials, and traffic. Even before the oil crisis in the Seventies everybody was eager to save energy. This was the main argument for recycling air in public buildings and apartment blocks, sometimes without filtration, so that indoor pollution accumulated and became seriously aggravated. This has led to concern among hygienists about the health effects of this practice. In more recent years large international conferences have been held where specialists have exchanged results from research in this area. The United States and Scandinavia have been pioneers in this, but a gradual realization of the problem has occurred all over the world. Today, as much as 50 per cent of all buildings in the civilized world are regarded as suffering from deficient ventilation, and the many complex problems of indoor air have been dubbed the 'sick building syndrome'.

Indoor air is consciously seen as a cause of decreased well-being and bad health among people who spend their time in it, and researchers have sought to prove that in the work place the cost of absenteeism and sick leave is ten times as expensive to the employer as would be the cost of proper ventilation. Specialists estimate that employees in offices and other work places in sick buildings have a lowered productivity and an increased absence rate. Twenty to 30 per cent of interviewed employees have felt the impact of the sick-building syndrome, usually a function of low-quality indoor air from insufficient ventilation and bad filtration.

The most frequently examined factors in recent years are radon and environmental tobacco smoke, volatile organic and inorganic substances from walls ('concrete sweat') and floor coverings, ozone from printers and other electric machines. Other factors focused upon are artificial light, illumination and heat radiation, radiation from electronic equipment (computers), noise and vibrations, temperature and humidity, as well as static electricity. Finally, there is increasing interest in bacteria, fungi, and fungal spores found in the air, especially where the air is recycled. But it's also important to consider the outdoor air – and the impact of nearby roads and motorways, car parks, basements, and factories: 'fresh air' coming in is no fresher than that of the outdoor environment.

The estimate is that a good ventilation system should be able to maintain the temperature between 20°C and 23°C, and an air humidity of between 30 and 60 per cent.

Sick buildings cause a series of vague but tangible symptoms among many of those who spend a lot of time inside the buildings. The symptoms are unlikely to be due to single factors, but to several factors combined, and they are given different weights by different people, that is, they are subjective and individual, and are, moreover, difficult to measure. These symptoms are phenomena such as discomfort, heavy breathing, irritation of eyes, nose, larynx, and skin, dryness of mucous membranes, sore throat, coughing, headache, drowsiness, and nausea. Confirmation of the diagnosis of sick-building syndrome is that the symptoms disappear when you leave the building in question.

The victims, who are as fresh as daisies and as fit as fiddles in their spare time and at weekends, are of course suspected by those responsible for the environment in the building of being hypochondriacs, lazy and work-shy. The whole problem, they say, comes from a lack of working morale. It is of great importance to solve the problem of how to measure the respective factors. Without this, we only have the major health repercussions – Pontiac fever, Legionnaire's disease, allergic rhinitis – to work with.

We will now deal with some of the most frequently studied

indoor pollution factors, but without maintaining those to be necessarily the most significant in all cases. There are, moreover, still many studies underway in this area, precisely because of a lack of knowledge.

Among potential chemical factors are carbon dioxide, carbon monoxide, nitric oxide, sulphur dioxide, volatile organic substances, mineral fibres, and radon (the radioactive gas that seeps into buildings and accumulates there, permanently radiating alpha-rays). Many of these substances influence health.

ETS, the contribution of tobacco to indoor air pollution, is the only factor that can be seen and smelled, and therefore it has been proclaimed an essential pollution problem. At any rate, it can be considered an excellent indicator of the efficiency of the ventilation. In reality, however, concentrations of nicotine (and cotinine, the only specific tracer of tobacco) have been measured in office workers, but at levels so low that they are approaching the lower limits of detection. As emphasized by the Brussels Convention in February 1989, no differences were found in concentrations of smoke particles, carbon monoxide, or carbon dioxide between non-smoking areas getting recycled air from smoking areas and those getting fresh air.

The methods of measuring the biological impact of tobacco smoke in the environment are not well defined and not very accurate. The epidemiological association of ETS and lung cancer has not been proven, and this is hardly surprising since the dose is so slight and the calculations can be dominated by other unknown contributory factors as well as 'a subjective, non-provable tendency to confirm the existing anti-smokers attitudes' (Brussels Convention).

The health effect of radon has also been under intense debate and is the subject of great disagreement. Experiments on animals have shown a relationship between radon radiation and lung cancer, and workers in uranium mines have also exhibited an increased risk of lung cancer because of the higher radon exposure. There is a lot of disagreement as to how to transfer these experiences to sick buildings, not least because the presence of radon in buildings is possibly due more to geographical location than to ventilation.

More than a hundred volatile organic substances have been found in indoor air. Formaldehyde and methylene chloride can be determined precisely, but contributions from building materials, furniture glue, detergents, pesticides, paint, and solvents are often quite complex – and can include well-known carcinogens. The concentration of these volatile substances has been measured at (under certain circumstances) eighty times higher than in outdoor air. PVC materials, for instance, give off considerable amounts of phenol and other organic substances with physiological effects for a long time after manufacture. Variations are, however, considerable and it is difficult to generalize.

Less volatile organic substances are also liberated from building materials, and accumulate in considerable concentrations on textiles, plastic coatings, and, especially, cotton fabrics. Contributing to the cocktail are inorganic substances, such as asbestos and mineral wool. But the constant development of new substances, glues, paints, diluents, detergents, and so on, demands a higher degree of cooperation between technicians and producers. And again, too little is known. It is, however, credible that people are influenced by many different substances, of which a number have been shown to increase health risks, while practically nothing is known about many others.

Carbon monoxide is probably the dominant indoor pollutant. Contributing to this are heaters, stoves, fireplaces, outdoor car traffic, and – not least – car parks below buildings. Even people contribute in a modest way. Modern buildings, which are highly insulated, without chimneys, without the facility to open windows (because it disturbs thermostats), and with recycled ventilation, are especially prone to carbon monoxide problems. Acute cases of life-threatening carbon monoxide poisoning have also occurred in old buildings heated by stoves where sooted pipes and chimneys have led to defective air-flow out of the stove.

Biological pollution is caused predominantly by people. Each person gives off heat, humidity, odours, sweat, scales, dandruff and hair, as well as dirt from clothing. Other organisms contribute – commonly fungi, bacteria, and dust mites. Many people think that these are actually responsible for the sick-building syndrome. On a material level, it has been found that 34 per cent of all sick buildings are contaminated by fungi and fungal spores, 9 per cent by bacteria, and in only 4 per cent can a contribution from ETS be found. Paradoxically, it doesn't help to increase ventilation because polluted ventilation channels and filters are frequently the source of bacterial and fungal pollution (this does not include ETS, of course).

Bacteria as well as fungi are frequent sources of infectious diseases, and have caused unpleasant epidemics among staff working in polluted buildings. Mites in house dust seem to be inexterminable, and they infest many residences, thriving in carpets and floor coverings, and are considered a primary problem all over the industrialized world. Of all cases of allergy ascribed to house dust, 99 per cent are due to mite excrement, which is proven to be allergenic. House dust mites live everywhere, in cushions, pillows, eiderdowns, blankets, clothing, curtains, and cracks. To fight this problem, cleaning with benzyl-benzoate and DDT is recommended. But this would contribute significantly to the sick-building syndrome, and to the strain on the indoor environment, perhaps even increase the cancer risk – who knows?

But, of course, it is much easier to forget the whole thing and concentrate all efforts on intense campaigns against tobacco smokers. As long as it is possible to make good people and authorities believe the importance of that. . . .

12

About Biology and Common Sense

In the course of human history, there has not been a generation less marked by disease than ours in modern developed countries. The standard of housing is generally high, hygiene is good, food is abundant, and physical demands of work are low. Wild animals and micro-organisms are kept in check with the help of technology, and the average life expectancy is extremely high. For men it is about seventy-two years, for women seventy-eight years (Danish figures).

Life expectancy for people having reached the age of fifty is twenty-five more years for men (i.e. seventy-five years), thirty for women (till the age of eighty). Acute diseases affect very small numbers and do not characterize modern life. The diseases we suffer from are chronic and progress slowly. What typifies our daily lives are anxieties, headaches, muscle pains, constipation, loss of hair, sex problems, tiredness, sleeplessness, irritation, being overweight – symptoms from the borderland of disease, rather more the results of stress, boredom, and the foolish conduct of life.

Considering that disease is so rare, and death occurs so late in life, it is strange that health problems ('health') and precautions to postpone death so dominate our consciousness.

Nearly all popular magazines and all daily newspapers carry copy on health risks and offer regular columns with health advice. Clothing, food recipes, rules of conduct, diets, training programmes, natural medicine, hygiene and how to take care of your body take up a lot of space. It has become a well-paid business to sell health in many forms to the people. And everybody can (and wants to) give good advice about what is healthy and unhealthy – at the moment. The scientific documentation is often scanty or non-existent. In spite of this, however, fashions change and at any time everybody is ready with advice, often mixed with a little moralizing.

One wonders why young people who can look forward to many years of life in good order and more mature people who can expect to survive until they reach eighty, bother themselves so intensely with all this stuff. Why do people put themselves through deprivation and all sorts of unpleasant procedures through so long a life – to gain a problematic survival of a few months more. But that is, nevertheless, what many people do. They devalue a long life to make it last even longer. . . .

Limits to health

Considering the fact that for so many people their last years are dull, powerless, poverty-stricken, lonely, or boring, it is inexplicable that they are so concerned with living long instead of living well.

The survival of the organism depends on the maintenance of a number of internal balances, collectively called the homeostasis. The homeostasis is regulated within narrow limits, by a balance of liquids, cell function, heart activity, function of kidneys, lungs and liver. In youth, most of the organs have perhaps ten times more capacity than is necessary to handle ordinary demands. This reserve capacity allows even damaged and stressed organs to manage to restore the homeostasis, if it is disturbed by external influences.

But with the advance of age, the reserves are diminished. Measurements of organ capacity through life show an almost linear decline, starting at the age of thirty and being roughly halved every eighth year – until there is no reserve in hand to help, when even a small disturbance of the homeostasis occurs.

Modern man who is not exposed, as were previous generations, to famine, cold, injuries, and severe infections, generally has reserves to restore the homeostasis to an advanced age. But the reserve capacity is diminished, so for him, too, even small disturbances become difficult to repair, in the end.

Figure 9: Speed of healing compared with patient's age, for a wound 40 cm^2 in area

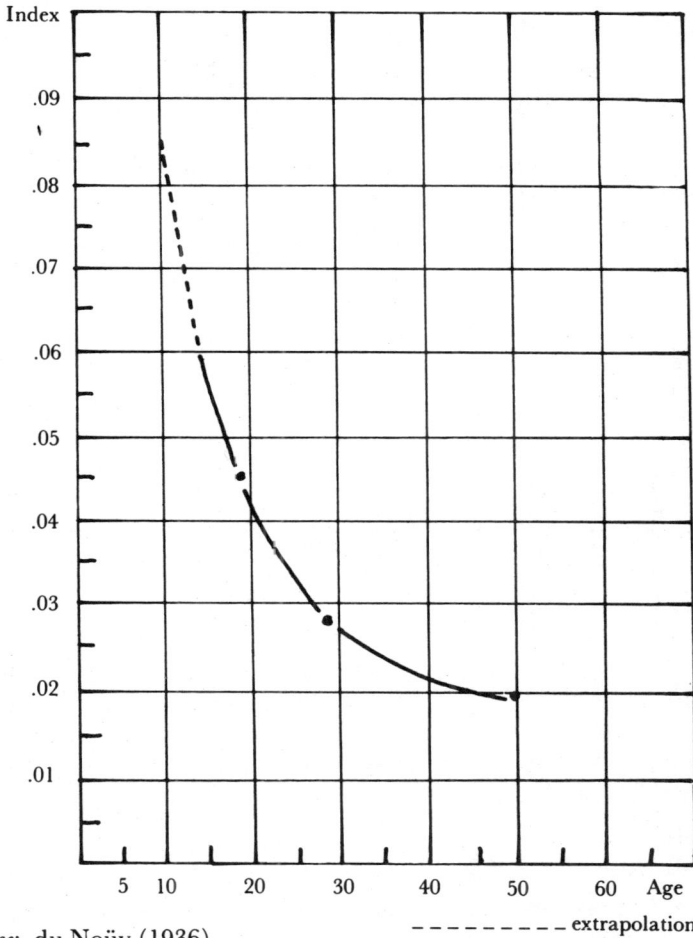

Source: du Noüy (1936)

Lecomte du Noüy has shown this by measuring the healing of wounds at various ages (Figure 9), and has taken the pace of healing as a reasonably general expression of biological activity. An eight-year-old heals a wound in ten days, a forty-year-old takes thirty-five days to heal a similar wound. The capacity to

Figure 10: How physiological functions diminish with age

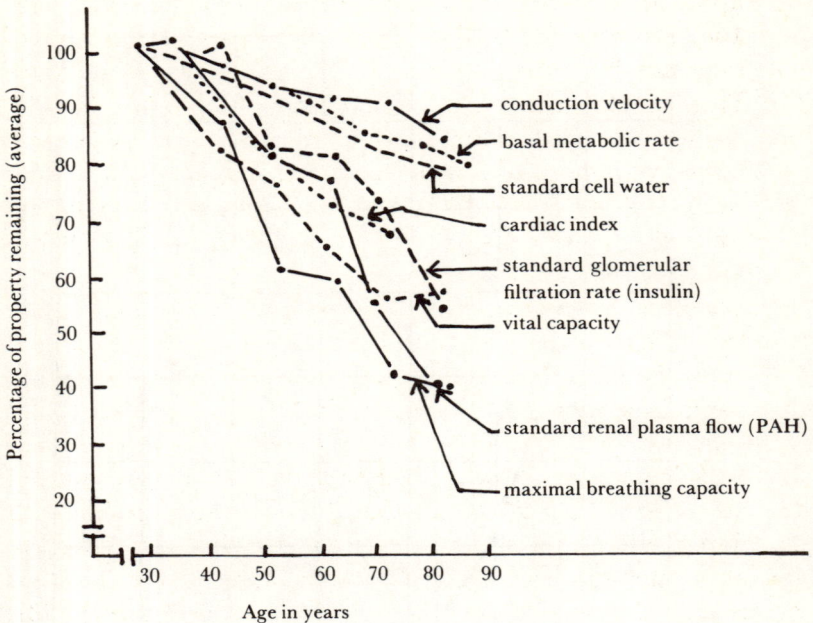

Source: Rudman (1987)

repair attrition and decay declines, and in the end vanishes. The homeostasis is broken, and the individual dies.

This phenomenon may also be seen in Figure 10 which shows the level of certain measurable physiological functions (metabolism, ability to coordinate, contents of liquid in cells, function of kidneys, lung capacity, and so on) at different ages. The condition of aging is obvious.

Up to the age of sixty ordinary stresses will be compensated for, but as vital functions decline, between seventy and eighty it becomes a matter of chance when stresses exceed the reserves, so that the system cannot cope. Similarly, chance will decide what kind of stress it will be. Death arrives, perhaps without any demonstrable cause, because the reserves are fully drained, and the homeostasis cannot be sustained. If death must have a reason, it finds one. The older we get, the more incidental is the cause of death.

Graphs can be drawn showing the death rates at different ages from the most common fatal diseases, giving us an impression of how mortality from each of those is increasing with age (Figure 11). They are, however, parallel, more or less. (Notice that the scale shown here is logarithmic, which means that every vertical interval corresponds to a scale ten times larger. 1–10 – next interval 10–100, next 100–1000, and so on, so that the gradients in advanced age are considerably steeper than that which immediately meets the eye.)

Acute disease is no longer a major medical problem for us. At the beginning of this century injuries and acute diseases were still important death causes. Tuberculosis, syphilis, rheumatic fever, smallpox, stomach infections, diphtheria, tetanus, polio, and simple pneumonia were the most frequent threats to the health of children and adults alike. Better nutrition, housing, hygiene, refuse disposal and purification of water, together with inoculation and antibiotics have caused a decline in the relative mortality rate of infectious diseases from more than 30 per cent to less than 2 per cent. Now the picture is different (Fig. 13). Chronic diseases are now to blame for more than 80 per cent of all deaths, and they arrive late: arteriosclerosis (including cerebral haemorrhage and cardiac thrombosis), arthritis, senile diabetes, lung changes and cancer are diseases of advanced age.

Characteristic of these diseases is that many of them have a long course, some of them start very early in life. It is often a matter of semantics whether to call arthrosis a disease or a natural consequence of attrition during life. A matter of words when to say that a disease started – yes, some may claim that degenerative diseases and wear and tear start at birth.

Experience from autopsies also teaches us that many of these conditions do not actually share the responsibility for death. Some of them have not even had time to manifest themselves, although they may have been developing over a long period. It may then look as if death is incidentally due to senescent diabetes, so that the cerebral arteriosclerosis and the vasoconstricted heart and the unrecognized cancer in the pancreas never

Figure 11: Deaths by age for varied conditions – including cancers

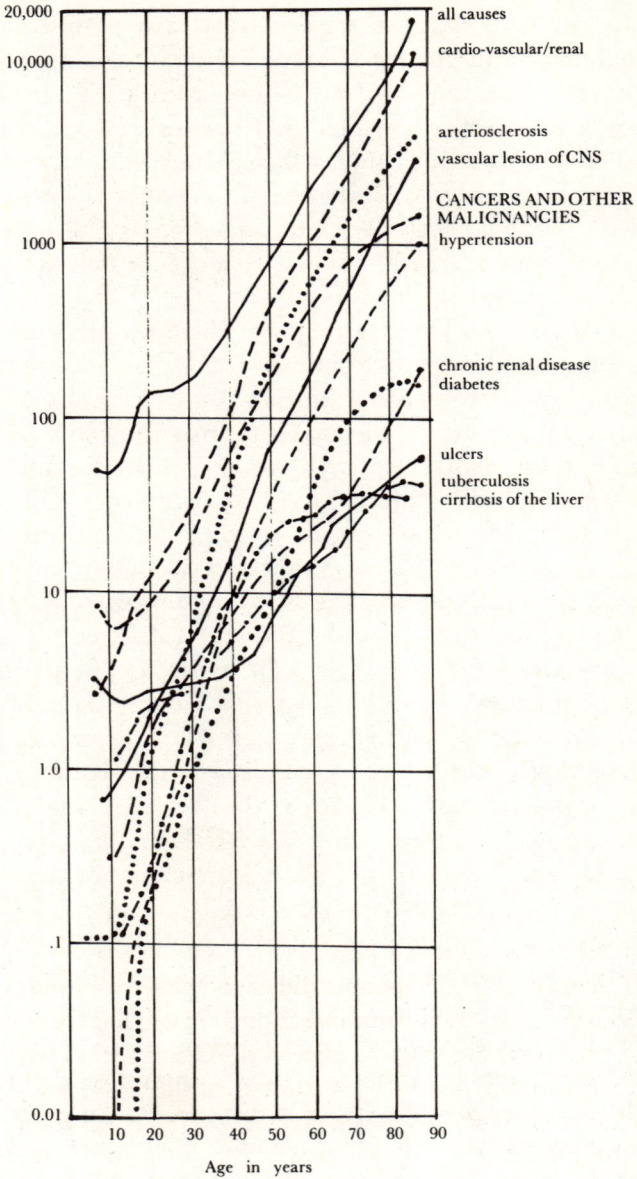

Source: Rudman (1987)

Figure 12:   Causes of death 1940 and 1980

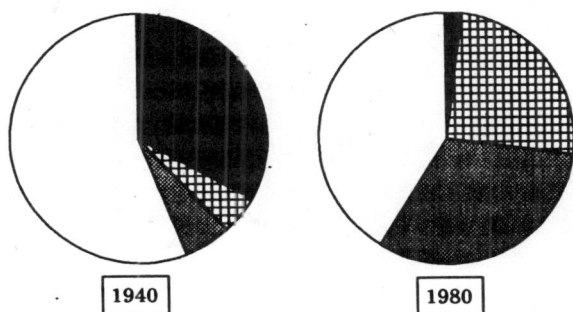

Note: the pie charts show how causes of death have changed between
1940 and 1980. Black = infectious diseases; hatching = cancers; dots = heart disease; white = accidents and all other
causes

had time to get their share. Or as if a heart attack in time
stopped the diabetes and made the cancer uninteresting. Or as if
some other chronic diseases were progressing slowly enough for
the cancer to have time to develop and claim the cause of death.

The gist of this explanation is that such processes progress
slowly with advancing age, and that some of them never have
time to show themselves and affect the homeostasis or mark the
individual's life before death arrives. And that the gain of being
spared one thing, at an advanced age, invariably abandons one
to the mercy of another. If then we should happen to avoid lung
cancer by abstaining from smoking, we would just die of cerebral
haemorrhage or something else.

A little less than 60,000 people die each year in Denmark. Fifty
years ago, one third died from infections, 5 per cent from cancer,
6 per cent from cardiovascular diseases. Around 1940 we got the
potent medicaments against infections, sulphonamides, penicil-
lin, the 'mycins – and infections as a cause of death fell to 2 per
cent of the total.

Figure 13:   Age at death

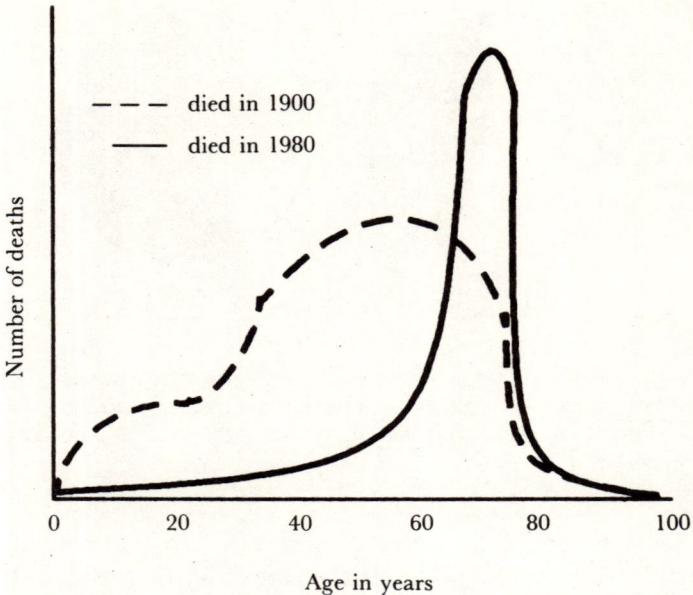

Age in years

Limits to life

After that, the average life expectancy did not increase very much and as people no longer died from infections, they had to die from something else. The share of cancer became 25 per cent, and that of cardiovascular diseases 32 per cent.

In 1936 if you were a man aged fifty you could expect to survive for another 23.6 years, which meant a total duration of life of 73.6 years. In 1987 you could expect less than two years longer, just twenty-five years.

Mice have a shorter life than dogs, dogs have a shorter life than humans. However much they adhere to all the rules of good health – whatever the fashion may be – following diets, having inoculations, jogging, humans rarely live to be a hundred years old. The current assumption is that average life expectancy will not exceed eighty-five years (Figure 13).

Figure 14: Age at death for those born in 1900 compared with predicted age at death for those born in 1980

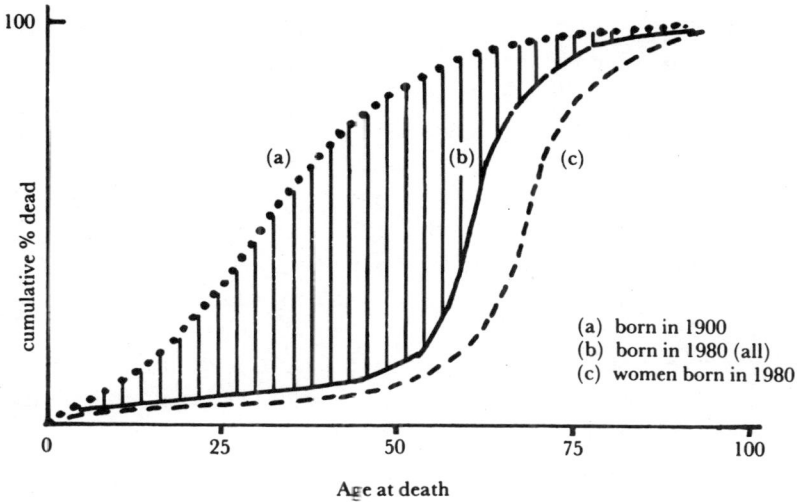

Note: in 1900 (a) people died at all ages but in 1980 (b) most can expect to die in old age. Women today (c) have the best chance

A cell has a capacity for division, on which growth and repair depend. Human fibroblasts seem to be able to manage a total of 50 divisions, whereafter growth stops, divisions cease, and the cells die. This happens for humans under ideal living conditions at between eighty and eighty-five years. The number of cell divisions seem to be specific for each species, mice have fewer, dogs more. No matter how we behave, it does not seem possible to change this circumstance.

The natural limit of survival can also be found in another way. The solid line in Figure 14 shows that even after eliminating acute diseases, the modern average duration of life is unlikely to exceed eighty-five years. A comparison with the age of arrival of death in the early 1900s (dotted line) demonstrates the difference between then and now: most people now die at a mature age.

At the beginning of the century life expectancy at birth was about forty-six years. It increased by 0.33 years each year until the 1940s. For 65-year-old people life expectancy was seventy-seven and the increase only 0.05 years each year. If you draw the curves they cross at the age of eighty-two.

In the 1980s the increase in life expectancy from birth (where it was about seventy-three years) was still 0.33 years per year, but the change in life expectancy at age sixty-five had increased to 0.12 years per year. These two curves would cross at a life expectancy of eighty-five years in the year 2018 (de Fries).

If we try to project this change into the future, it turns out that until the year 2025 we get, through flattening of the curve, a constant approach to an age a little over eighty-five, which must be considered the maximum attainable average life expectancy (de Fries).

In the year 1900 people in Northern Europe died thirty-eight years 'too soon' (sooner than our theoretically calculated life expectancy). In 1950 they died seventeen years 'too soon', in 1980 only twelve years 'too soon'. In 1980 a woman would die only seven years 'too soon'. And three of these years will be due to accidents. We can safely say that the benefits of medicine and social improvements from now on can only result in small changes in the average life span. Figure 14 shows that even intense medical and preventive efforts can do little to make the curve steeper. The shaded area shows the gains obtained from the successful fight against acute diseases since 1900.

What are the implications of all this for the fight against cancer? Suppose there were to be a solution to the mystery of cancer and it was no longer a cause of death. Täuber estimated that this would mean an increase in average life expectancy of a maximum of 14 months: other demographers have made it much less. This is not exactly what some people would like us to think – it is not in the vicinity of eternal life. Fortunately. Because while politicians and the authorities take great care that we do not die from smoking tobacco, they express great concern about the increasing number of old people in our society. How are we supposed to cope with all those?

It would be practical if we decided what is most worrying: that people die – or that people do not die.

Common sense . . .

There is much to indicate that, no matter what we do, human
life expectancy is biologically limited, and that the limit (statistically) lies somewhere between seventy-five and eighty-five years.
A car used normally has a lifetime of twelve to fourteen years,
dependent more (as with humans) on maintenance and care
than on use. If the coachwork does not rust away, then the clutch
breaks down, or the gear box. Or the pistons. Or the brakes. Or
the electrical system is finished. Repairs and replacements can
be made. But eventually the decay becomes too extensive for the
owner to handle.

The same thing happens to the human organism. If the joints
are not worn out, then the brain is. Or the eye lens. Or the heart
or the kidneys. Or the circulatory system. What it is, is not
interesting. Death will have a cause, this one or that one. And if
we do not die from cancer, we die in time from something else.

On the basis of this, the fierce and expensive crusade against
tobacco seems a bit senseless. Apart from the fact that the
connection between smoking tobacco and contracting cancer or
cardiovascular disease is so uncertain.

Considering that 82 per cent of all cancer deaths hit people
over sixty years of age, where mortality is steeply increasing, one
could be tempted to regard cancer not as a disease – but simply
as a cause of death.

13

A Little Philosophy of Life (and Death)

The doctor is sitting at the bedside. Yes, the doctor still sits at bedsides – in underdeveloped countries where there is quite a lot of illness and people die early. His patients in the beds are often children, young people. The middle aged – the ones that get that far – are tough and not so often acutely ill: and the old people regard frailty and decay as inevitable.

The doctor wants to cure his patients. He seeks means for this end. All his efforts are concentrated on fighting diseases: on a greater understanding of them, on better remedies against them. This is his function, as it has been through the centuries.

That is the way it was in the more developed countries until fifty years ago. Now it is different. The doctor is still sitting at the bedside, but his patients in the beds have become old people, and most often they suffer from the chronic diseases of age, demanding more care than treatment.

But the doctor doesn't seem to have noticed that the patient in the sick-bed at his side has become old. He still fights diseases, concentrates on symptoms and causes, feels obliged to cure the patient, free him from disease, save his life. Cure his age. . . .

Responding to tradition, he flings himself at the eighty-year-old patient whose heart has stopped; intubates, starts heart massage, sends for the respirator. Blindly and without ulterior motives he operates on cancer tumours, renews organs, starts intensive treatment, restores fluid balance. His treatment is so skilful and meticulous that many people are scared and decide well ahead of time that they want to be allowed to die reasonably peacefully and without too much officious meddling.

Whether the patient is young or old, cheerful or miserable, the

129

doctor works to save his life. Of course, he does not look askance at the age of his patient; should he treat less well because his patient is old; would he treat less actively, less hopefully? If a child dies, it loses many years of its life expectancy. But although average duration of life in European countries is calculated to be between seventy and eighty years, everybody has, when growing older, an expected life span left. The eighty-year-old has statistically six to seven years. Are those the years the doctor is fighting to save, for the eighty-five-year-old, the ninety-year-old?

Few ask what kind of years we'll enjoy as old people. Few notice that the suicide rate among men over sixty-five in Denmark is twice as high as that of the average population. This does not affect the doctor, although it raises the question of the quality of many people's last years. There is no professional tradition among physicians to be interested in this. It belongs to the realm of social workers and politicians.

More and more diseases are due to attrition and decay of organs, for which there is no particularly effective treatment. That is why it becomes more and more the interest of physicians to prevent such processes, prevent the diseases. While we know quite a lot about the nature of diseases, about their causes and treatment, our knowledge of the wearing down of the mechanism by life is very loose. Physicians tend to offer positive assertions and good advice that is at worst wrong, at best useless, and of minor importance for the progress towards death.

Nowadays, physicians talk a lot about health, about the preservation of health, how we should live, eat, and drink (and how not!), without actually knowing anything concrete about the matter. Physicians often and gladly interfere in the conduct of their patients and their habits. The noble purpose is to save good people from disease and early death, even from late death, from any kind of death. Isn't it then a bit strange not to take notice of the conditions and quality of life in the closing years, those years they so beautifully fight to preserve for their patients. . . .

This is actually what we do. What doctors do. As a consequence of specialization, lung specialists react against the diagnosis lung disease, heart specialists against death from heart disease. Their work focuses on the diseases of their specialty, and on

reducing mortality from these causes. Let people die of diabetes
or senile dementia, says the chest man. But not of lung disease!

Cancer patients may never hear how many people die from
disseminated sclerosis, and how they die (or live with it). Even
though it might share the body with the sclerosis, cancer is the
only thing that is important to the patient. And as society cannot
have the same attitude to cancer as cancer patients and cancer
treatment staff, an organization is founded with the purpose of
creating interest, procuring means for treatment and scientific
research in precisely this disease.

Powerful organizations are collecting money and lobbying for
cancer, others for lung diseases, others again for heart diseases,
epilepsy, diabetes, blindness, sclerosis. Each disease has its organization, its financial means, its managers, its institutes, its
scientists, and its therapeutic domains. Some of them are almost
small states within the state, fighting among themselves in a
bitter contest about influence and means.

The Society for Fighting Cancer and its servants are preoccupied with reducing the incidence of the disease; in all humility, of
course, in order to bring about the total extinction of cancer
diseases, and elimination of cancer as a cause of death.

Now suppose this organization succeeded in its aims and
discovered how to avoid cancer – and so did those other organizations with their respective diseases. We would have this total
knowledge: how to avoid death. The question becomes: how to
obtain death – if there are no causes left. . . .

It would become a distinct problem – of what then are people
going to die? And the touching fact is that nobody has paused to
consider the philosophical (or the demographic) consequence of
this. Would it be eternal life if nobody died at all? And what
would the consequences of this be for our society, and for our
existence on the whole? Do none of these restlessly working
problem solvers think about this, contemplate it at their conferences. . . ?

It seems that physicians have been betrayed by their lack
of professional philosophy, as patients are betrayed by their
lack of philosophy of life. Our only guideline is: general protest
against dying. Not fear of being dead (which is actually often

people's wish). But despite the fact that the mystery of existence behind the gate of death has preoccupied all cultures, our only concern is the fear of the process itself: dying. Our plea to the doctor then becomes this specific one: Give me something so that I do not feel anything, so that I get out by the backdoor if it actually has to be. But preferably not at all.

What happens, then, to the philosophical aspect of eternal life, eternal youth? Is it ever being contemplated? And if it is being contemplated, how is this eternal life to be lived, on what conditions . . .?

Paradoxically, physicians, of all people, are those who have demonstrated that appalling conditions give rotten lives. More than a hundred years ago, Robert Kock demonstrated that the tuberculosis bacillus was the cause of a disease that decimated the populations of the civilized world. But experience taught us that not until we had better hygiene, proper housing standards, and decent food was it possible to stop the ravages of disease, years before potent antibacterials to help fight infection were found. It more than suggests that this disease is not primarily a bacterial matter – but a social disease statistically dominating social groups living under bad conditions. This ought to lead to thoughts about why some can survive although they break all health directives, while others who obey them live a miserable, short, and illness-dominated life. Why can some people regale themselves with roast pork and crackling and stay in top form till they grow to ninety, others smoke merrily from dawn to dusk a whole long life through without any signs of lung symptoms – while others become sick of it? And some even without it . . .?

Wouldn't it be wise here to consider the simple socio-medical association between resources and stresses, and realize that individuals with a generally high level of resources to a great extent are invincible against the world's harassments and plagues – including tobacco. Forty-five years have now passed since Vagn Christensen demonstrated the connection between living quarters and children's sickliness. There are surely other social parameters with links to genuine, politically sensitive health issues, too. It is a well-known fact that knowledge of health – and strength to realize one's knowledge in one's daily life – go together with social status.

Hardships lead to bad eating habits, poor hygiene, and misuse of medicine, alcohol, and tobacco. And to low resistance towards any kind of diseases. I think it would be reasonable to remember this in connection with this debate. . . .

Why does a doctor's advice not include injunctions to get a decent residence, sensible nutrition, non-stressful work, not to become poor? Does this absolve us from making an effort to achieve better living conditions for those who are worst off, for doing something against pollution of air and water, against problems of refuse disposal, against the accumulation of poison everywhere in the industrialized world, against the stress from unhealthy jobs, noise and dust pollution, overpopulation in big cities, traffic nuisance, and industrial contamination, the consequences of fast food, bad housing, sick building syndromes, depressions, sleeplessness and fatigue due to stress, loneliness, unemployment, boredom . . .?

Why does the concern of doctors and authorities never include the basic resources of people – but only those stresses that are not the responsibility of our societies? Each and every health campaign and all good advice and instructions are concerned with what the individual himself may do to survive in a mistreated, stressed, and chaotic world. Concern for the environment and our fellow creatures goes as far as whales. Where humans are concerned, responsibility is privatized and becomes their own. You must never. . . . You shall always. . . . If the air has been destroyed and polluted by poisons and dust, you must hold your breath! And if you don't, the consequences are your own responsibility.

Can we forget all these circumstances and only concentrate on living up to health instructions, for instance give up smoking? Can we really believe that world health depends on that?

Can it really be true that the key solution to global pollution lies in fighting tobacco smoking? Are we supposed to believe that and forget everything else, the death of forests, the hole in the ozone layer, the lead poisoning. . . .

Will we really solve the essential world health problems before the year 2000 by stopping tobacco smoking? Will we increase the life expectancy of the world population simply by eliminating tobacco? Will we improve people's quality of life by forbidding them to smoke tobacco if they happen to like it . . .?

The answer can be read every day in the newspaper. But the facts whisper in the wind.

References

The Harmful Effects of Smoking

ALTAMURA, R. F., 'Children, pets and disease', *J. Am. Osteopathic Assn*, 1982, 81(5): 334–40.

AUERBACH, O. *ET AL.*, 'Histologic types of lung cancer in relation to smoking habits', *Chest*, 1975, 67(4): 382–7.

BLOT, N. J. & FRAUMENI, J. F., 'Geographic patterns of lung cancer: Industrial correlations', *Am. J. Epidem.*, 1976, 103: 539–50.

BONHAM, G. S. & WILSON, R. W., 'Children's health in families with cigarette smokers', *Am. J. Public Health*, 1981, 71(3): 290–3.

BRITTON, M., 'Diagnostic errors discovered at autopsy', *Acta Med. Scand.*, 1974, 196: 203–10.

BRITTON, M., 'Clinical diagnosis: Experience from 383 autopsied cases', *Acta Med. Scand.*, 1974, 196: 211–19.

BURCH, P., 'Smoking and lung cancer: The problem of inferring causes', *J. Roy. Stat. Soc.*, 1978, 141(4): 437–77.

CAMERON, H. M. & MCGOOGAN, E., 'A prospective study of 1152 hospital autopsies: Analysis of inaccuracies in clinical diagnoses and their significance', *J. Path.*, 1981, 133/4: 285–300.

DOLL, R. & HILL, A. B., 'Lung cancer and other causes of death in relation to smoking: A second report on the mortality of British doctors', *Brit. Med. J.*, 1956, 2: 1071–81.

DOLL, R. & HILL, A. B., 'Mortality in relation to smoking – ten years' observations of British doctors', *Brit. Med. J.*, 1964, 1: 1399–1410.

EHRLICH, D. *ET AL.*, 'Some factors affecting the accuracy of cancer diagnosis', *J. Chron. Dis.*, 1975, 28/7–8: 359–64.

FACCINI, J. M., 'The role of histopathology in evaluation of risk of lung cancer from environmental tobacco smoke', *Exp. Path.*, 1989, 37(1–4): 177–80.

FEINSTEIN, A. R. & WELLS, G. K., 'Cigarette smoking and lung cancer:

The problems of detecting bias in epidemiologic rates of disease', *Trans. Assoc. Am. Physicians*, 1974, 87: 180–5.

FISHER, R. A., *Smoking: The Cancer Controversy, Some Attempts to Assess the Evidence*. Oliver & Boyd, London, 1959.

GITTELSOHN, A. & SENNING, J., 'Studies on the reliability of vital and health records: I. Comparison of cause of death and hospital record diagnoses', *Am. J. Public Health*, 1979, 69/7: 680–9.

HAMMOND, E. C., 'Smoking in relation to the death rates of one million men and women', in Haenszel (ed.), *Epidemiological Approaches to the Study of Cancer and other Chronic Diseases*, National Cancer Institute Monograph 19, US DHEW, US PHS, NCI, 1966.

HOLST, P. A. *ET AL.*, 'For debate: Pet birds as an independent risk factor for lung cancer', *Brit. Med. J.*, 1988, 297: 1319–21.

LEHRER, S. B. *ET AL.*, 'Tobacco smoke sensitivity: A result of allergy?' *Annals of Allergy*, 1986, 56: 369–81.

LOCK, W., *Die Konstanz der Gesamtkrebsmortalität in den Altersgruppen. Ursachen und Perspektive*. Urban & Vogel, München, 1988.

OWNBY, D. R. & MCCULLOUGH, J., 'Passive exposure to cigarette smoke does not increase allergic sensitisation in children', *J. Allergy and Clin. Immun.*, 1988, 82/4: 634–8.

PATTY, F. A. (ED.), *Industrial Hygiene and Toxicology*, 2nd ed., Wiley, New York, 1958.

STEVENS, R. G. & MOOLGAVKAR, S. H., 'A cohort analysis of lung cancer and smoking in British males', *Am. J. Epidemiol.*, 1984, 119/4: 624–41.

US DEPT OF HEALTH, EDUCATION & WELFARE. *Smoking and Health: A Report of the Surgeon General*, DHEW Publ. 79–50066, 1979.

WELLS, C., 'Primary bronchiogenic carcinoma: Incidence, pathogenesis and diagnosis', *Am. Otol. Rhinol. Laryngol.*, 1934, 43: 561–71.

WILSON, M. J. & LEE, P. N. (EDS.), *Tobacco Consumption in Various Countries*, Tobacco Research Council, Research Paper No. 6, London, 1975.

ZACHAU–CHRISTIANSEN, B., *Development during the First Year of Life*, Helsingör, 1972.

The Beneficial Effects of Smoking, and Why We Smoke

AARRO, L. E. *ET AL.*, 'Health behaviour in schoolchildren: A WHO cross-national survey', *Health Promotion*, 1986, 1(1): 17–33.

BODDEWYN, J. J. (ED.), *Juvenile Smoking – Initiation and Advertising*, International Advertising Association, New York, 1989.

EDWARDS, J. A. *ET AL.*, 'Evidence of more rapid stimulus evaluation following cigarette smoking', *Addictive Behaviour*, 1985, 10(2): 113–26.

GEORGJEDDE, A. & VOSS, T., *Drik eller Druk*, Borgen, 1982.

GILBERT, G. D. *ET AL.*, 'Effects of smoking nicotine on anxiety, heart rate and lateralization of EEG during a stressful movie', *Psychophysiology*, 1989, 26(3): 311–20.

HASENFRATZ, M. *ET AL.*, 'Can smoking increase attention in rapid information processing during noise? Electrocortical, physiological and behavioral effects', *Psychopharmacology*, 1989, 98(1): 75–80.

HEIMSTRA, N. W. *ET AL.*, 'The effects of deprivation of cigarette smoking on psychomotor performance', *Ergonomics*, 1980, 23/11: 1047–55.

HOFSTETTER, A. *ET AL.*, 'Increased 24-hour energy expenditure in cigarette smokers', *New Engl. J. Med.*, 1986, 314(2): 79–82.

REMOND, A. & IZARD, C., *Electrophysiological Effects of Nicotine*, Elsevier, Amsterdam, 1979.

ROYAL SOCIETY OF CANADA. *Tobacco, Nicotine and Addiction*, 1989.

RUDMAN, D., 'Nutrition and fitness in elderly people', *Am. J. Clin. Nutr.*, 1987, 49: 1090–8.

TOLLISON, R. D. (ED.), *Smoking and Society: Towards a More Balanced Assessment*, Lexington Books, Massachusetts, 1986.

US DEPARTMENT OF HEALTH AND HUMAN SERVICES. *A Report of the Surgeon General. The Health Consequences of Smoking. Nicotine Addiction.* DHSS Publ. 88–8406, 1988.

VAN–RAAIJ, W. J., 'The effect of marketing communication on the initiation of juvenile smoking', in Van-Raaij, W. J. (ed.), *The Impact of Tobacco Advertising: A Special Report. Internat. J. Advertising*, Cassell, 1990.

VOSS, T. & ZIIRSEN, M., *Stofmisbrug – en samfundssygdom* Thaning & Appel, 1971.

WHAREN, J. *ET AL.*, 'Influence of cigarette smoking on body oxygen consumption', *Clin. Physiol.*, 1983, 3(1): 91.

WARBURTON, D. M. *ET AL.*, 'Facilitation of learning and state dependency with nicotine', *Psychopharmacology*, 1986, 89(1): 55–9.

WARBURTON, D. M., 'The puzzle of nicotine use', in Lader, M. H. (ed.), *The Psychopharmacology of Nicotine*, Oxford University Press, 1988, p27–49.

WARBURTON, D. M., 'Is nicotine use an addiction?' *The Psychologist*, 1989, 2(4): 166–70.

WESNES, K. & WARBURTON, D. M., 'The effects of cigarette smoking and nicotine tablets upon human attention', in Lader, M. H. (ed.) *The Psychopharmacology of Addiction*, Oxford University Press, 1988.

WESNES, K. & WARBURTON, D. M., 'Smoking, nicotine and human performance', *Pharmacol. & Ther.*, 1983, 21(2): 189–200.

WESNES, K. & WARBURTON, D. M., 'Effects of scopolamine and nicotine on human rapid information processing performance', *Psychopharmacology*, 1984, 82: 147–50.

WETTERER, A. & VON TROSCHKE, J., *Smoker Motivation: A Review of Contemporary Literature*, Springer Verlag, 1986.

WHO: EXPERT COMMITTEE ON DRUGS DEPENDENCE. *16th Report*. Tech. Rept Series 407, 1969.

WOODSON, P. P. *ET AL.*, 'Effects of nicotine on the visual evoked response', *Pharmacology, Biochemistry and Behaviour*, 1982, 17(5): 915–20.

What Substances have What Impact?

BANBURY REPORT 3. Gori, G. B. & Bock, F. G. (eds.). Cold Spring Harbor Lab., New York, 1980.

BELCHER, J. R., 'The changing pattern of bronchial carcinoma', *Brit. J. Dis. Chest*, 1987, 81(1): 87–95.

BLOT, W. J., 'Lung cancer and occupational exposures', in Hizzel, M. & Correa, P. (eds.), *Lung Cancer – Causes and Prevention*, Verlag Chemie Int. Inc, New Orleans, 1984.

BURCH, P. R., 'Smoking and lung cancer. The problem of interfering cause', *J. Stat. Soc. A.*, 1978, 141(4): 437–77.

GUERIN, M. R. *ET AL.*, 'The analysis of the particulate and vapour phases of tobacco smoke', in O'Neill, I. K. *et al.* (eds.), *Environmental Carcinogens*, vol. 9. *Passive Smoking*, IARC, Lyon, 1987.

HINDS, M. W. *ET AL.*, 'Differences in lung cancer risk from smoking among Japanese, Chinese and Hawaiian women in Hawaii', *Int. J. Cancer*, 1981, 27(3): 297–302.

HJERMANN, I. *ET AL.*, 'Effect of diet and smoking intervention on the incidence of coronary heart disease', *Lancet*, 1981, 2: 1303–10.

JENKINS, R. A. & GUERIN, M. R., 'General analytical considerations for the sampling of tobacco smoke', in O'Neill, I. K. *et al.* (eds.) *Environmental Carcinogens*, vol. 9. *Passive Smoking*. IARC, Lyon, 1987.

KEIL, U. & KUULASMAA, R. (EDS.), 'WHO MONICA Project', *Int. J. Epidemiol.*, 1989, 18 (Supplement 1): S46–S55.

LEAVERTON, P. E. *ET AL.*, 'Representatives of the Framingham risk model for coronary heart disease mortality. A comparison with a national cohort study', *J. Chron. Dis.*, 1987, 40(8): 775–84.

MACMAHON, S. *ET AL.*, 'Epidemiology: Blood pressure, stroke and coronary heart disease. Part 1', *Lancet*, 1990, 335: 765–74.

MCCORMICK, J. & SKRABANEK, P., 'Coronary heart diseases are not preventable by population interventions', *Lancet*, 1988, 2: 839–41.

MENOTTI, A. & SEOCARECCIA, F., 'Blood pressure, serum cholesterol and smoking habits predicting different manifestations of arteriosclerotic disease', *Acta Card,* 1987, 42(2): 91–102.

MÖLLER, K. O., *Farmakologi,* Busck, 1941.

MULTIPLE RISK FACTOR INTERVENTION TRIAL RESEARCH GROUP, 'Risk factor changes and mortality results', *J. Am. Med. Assoc.*, 1982, 248: 1468–77.

RAND, M. J. & THURAU, K. (EDS.) *The Pharmacology of Nicotine*, IRL Press, Oxford, 1987.

RAWBONE, R. G. *ET AL.*, 'The analysis of smoking parameters: Inhalation and absorption of tobacco smoke in studies on human smoking behaviour', in Thornton, R. E. (ed.), *Smoking Behaviour*, Longman, London, 1978.

RAWBONE, R. G., 'The act of smoking', in Cumming, G. & Bonsignore, G. (eds.), *Smoking and the Lung*, Plenum Press, London, 1984.

ROSE, G. *ET AL.*, 'UK heart disease prevention project. Incidence and mortality results', *Lancet*, 1983, 1: 1062–8.

SELTZER, C. C., 'Framingham study data and "established wisdom" about cigarette smoking and coronary heart disease', *J. Clin. Epidemiol.*, 1989, 42(8): 743–50.

SHY, C. M., 'Air pollution and lung cancer', in Hizzel, M. & Correa, P. (eds.), *Lung Cancer – Causes and Prevention*, Verlag Chemie Int. Inc, New Orleans, 1984.

SKRABANEK, P. & MCCORMICK, J., *Follies and Fallacies in Medicine*, Tarragon Press, Glasgow, 1989.

STERLING, T., 'Does smoking kill workers or working kill smokers?', *Int. J. Health Services*, 1978, 8(3): 437–52.

WALD, N. & FROGGATT, P., *Nicotine, Smoking and The Low Tar Programme*, Oxford University Press, 1989.

WHO EUROPEAN COLLABORATIVE GROUP, 'European collaborative trial of multi-factorial prevention of coronary heart disease: final report of the 6-year results', *Lancet*, 1986, 1: 869–72.

The Harmful Effects of Passive Smoking

ADLKOFER, F., *ET AL.*, 'Small airways dysfunction in passive smokers', *New Engl. J. Med.*, 1980, 303(7): 392.

AHLBORN, N. & ÜBERLA, K., 'Passive smoking and lung cancer: Reanalysis of Hirayama's data', in Perry, R. & Kirk, P. N. (eds.), *Indoor and Ambient Air Quality*, Selper, London, 1988.

ARONOW, W. J., 'Effects of passive smoking in angina pectoris', *New Engl. J. Med.*, 1980, 299(1): 21–4.

AVIADO, D. M., 'Health issues relating to "passive smoking"', in Tollison, R. D. (ed.), *Smoking and Society: Towards a More Balanced Assessment. Lexington Books*, Massachusetts, 1986.

ENSTROM, J. E. & GODLEY, F. H., 'Rising cancer mortality among nonsmokers', *J. Nat. Cancer Inst.*, 1979, 62(4): 755–60.

ENSTROM, J. E. & GODLEY, F. H., 'Cancer mortality among a representative sample of nonsmokers in the United States 1966–68', *J. Nat. Cancer Inst.*, 1980, 65(5): 1175–83.

FREEDMAN, A. P., 'Small airways dysfunction in passive smoking', *New Engl. J. Med.*, 1980, 303(7): 393.

FRIEDMAN, G. D. *ET AL.*, 'Prevalence and correlates of passive smoking', *Am. J. Public Health*, 1983, 73(4): 401–5.

GARFINKEL, L., 'Cancer mortality in nonsmokers: A prospective study by the American Society', *J. Nat. Cancer Inst.*, 1980, 65(5): 1169–73.

GARFINKEL, L. *ET AL.*, 'Time trends in lung cancer mortality among non-smokers and a note on passive smoking', *J. Nat. Cancer Inst.*, 1981, 66(6): 1061–6.

GARFINKEL, L. *ET AL.*, 'Involuntary smoking and lung cancer. A case-control study', *J. Nat. Cancer Inst.*, 1985, 75(3): 463–9.

HIRAYAMA, T., 'Non-smoking wives of heavy smokers have a higher risk of lung cancer', *Brit. Med. J.*, 1981, 282: 183–5.

HOUSE, R., *The Health Effects of Exposure to Tobacco Smoke*, Health Study Service, Ontario Min. of Labour, 1985.

HUBER, G. L., 'Small airways dysfunction in passive smokers', *New Engl. J. Med.*, 1980, 303(7): 392–3.

KILPATRICK, S. J., 'Chronic health effects of environmental tobacco smoke: A critique of the epidemiologic literature', *Objection to Committee on Passive Smoking, National Research Council*, Nat. Academy of Sciences, Wash. D.C. 1986.

LEE, P. N. *ET AL.*, 'Relationship of passive smoking to risk of lung cancer and other smoking-associated diseases', *Brit. J. Cancer*, 1986, 54: 97–105.

LEE, P. N., *Misclassification of Smoking Habits and Passive Smoking: A Review of the Evidence*, Springer-Verlag, 1988.

MCNICHOL, M. & TURNER, J. A., 'Oxygen uptake at the onset of angina pectoris: Effects of nicotine and carbon monoxide', *Clin. Science*, 1983, 65(3): 24.

MINTZ, M., 'FDA citing phony evidence', *The Washington Post*, 23 March 1983.

PETERSON, C., 'EPA probe criticizes a study used in air quality standard', *The Washington Post*, 7 June 1983.

O' NEILL, I. K. (ED.), *Environmental Carcinogens*, vol. 9: *Passive Smoking*, IARC, Lyon, 1987.

SCHNEIDER, B., 'What is risk and how can it be assessed', *Env. Technology*, 1990, 11: 585–98.

TRICHOPOULOS, D. *ET AL.*, 'Lung cancer and passive smoking', *Int. J. Cancer*, 1981, 27: 1–4.

US DEPARTMENT OF HEALTH EDUCATION AND WELFARE. *Smoking and Health. A Report of the Surgeon General*, DHEW Publ 79–50066, 1979.

US DEPARTMENT OF HEALTH AND HUMAN SERVICES. *The Health Consequences of Smoking: Cancer. A Report of the Surgeon General*, DHSS Publ 82–50179, 1982.

WHITE, J. R. & FROEB, H. E., 'Small airways dysfunction in non-smokers chronically exposed to tobacco smoke', *New Engl. J. Med.*, 1980, 302(13): 720–3.

Indoor Air

For those who want to read broadly or more specifically about the problems concerning tobacco smoke and environment, try this excellent introduction to the subject: TOLLISON, R. D., *Clearing the Air: Perspectives on Environmental Tobacco Smoke*, Lexington Books, Massachusetts, 1988.
A bit more detailed is the book edited by the same author: TOLLISON, R. D. (ED.). *Smoking and Society. Towards a More Balanced Assessment*, Lexington Books, Massachusetts, 1986.
PERRY, R. & KIRK, D. W. (EDS.). *Indoor and Ambient Air Quality*, Selper, London, 1988. This book contains a long series of specialist papers from all over the world collected and presented at a large London conference. Similar reports exist from a conference in Spain in 1989 and from a workshop in Geneva in 1983.
INFOTAB's concentrated *Environmental Tobacco Smoke*, 1986. *Tobacco Smoke and the Non-Smoker*, from The Tobacco Institute, Wash. D. C. 1987, is a rapidly read sober review of the whole problem, with numerous references.
There are also reviews of the medical and political considerations in WALD, N. & FROGGATT, D., *Nicotine, Smoking and The Low Tar Programme*, Oxford University Press, 1989.
You can find psychological accounts in WETTERER, A. & VON TROSCHKE,

J., *Smoker Motivation: A Review of Contemporary Literature*, Springer–Verlag, 1986.

We have also mentioned the WHO review by the International Agency for Cancer Research, Lyon, of the whole literature and all published papers on the subject up to November 1987 (more than 1,000 studies).

Those who are interested in very technical examinations of the Indoor Air problem can turn to *ASHRAE Standards* or subscribe to *Environmental Technology Letters* published by Selper, London, eds. Harrison & Lester, if they do not feel able to read the five volumes about Healthy Buildings published in Stockholm (Swedish Council for Building Research, 1988).

The whole field is very broad, with political and judicial aspects of a rather serious nature. But one can easily lose oneself in the subject, because these specific areas are quite exciting and in a way relevant for the assessment of the importance of tobacco on humans.

But as we said, the literature is prolific. And it is, to be sure, not all about tobacco.

BIEVA, C. J. *ET AL.*, 'Present and future of indoor air quality. Proceedings of the Brussels Conference, 14–16 Feb 1989', *Excerpta med Amsterdam*, 1989.

CARSON, J. R. & ERICKSON, A., 'Results from survey of environmental tobacco smoke in offices in Ottawa, Ontario', *Env. Techn. Letters*, 1988, 9: 501–8.

HUFF, D., *How to Lie with Statistics*, Harmondsworth, 1964.

JENKINS, R. A. & GUERIN, M. R., 'General analytical considerations for the sampling of tobacco smoke in indoor air', in O' Neill, I. K. (ed.). *Environmental Carcinogens*, vol. 9: *Passive Smoking*, IARC, Lyon, 1987.

LEE, P. N., *Misclassification of Smoking Habits and Passive Smoking: A Review of the Evidence*, Springer–Verlag, 1988.

LETZEL, H. *ET AL.*, 'Meta-analyses on passive smoking and lung cancer: effects of study selection and misclassification of exposure', *Env. Techn. Letters*, 1988, 9(6): 491–500.

HULKA, B. S. (CHAIRMAN) NATIONAL RESEARCH COUNCIL, US., *Environmental Tobacco Smoke: Measuring Exposures and Assessing Effects*. Nat. Academy Press, 1986.

PROCTOR, C. J., 'Analysis of the contribution of ETS to indoor air', in Perry, R. & Kirk, P. W. (eds.), *Indoor and Ambient Air Quality*, Proc. Indoor Amb. Air Quality Conf., Selper, London, 1988.

SCHWARTZ, S. L. & BALTER, N. J., 'ETS–lung cancer epidemiology: Supportability of misclassification and risk assumptions', *Env. Techn. Letters*, 1988, 9: 479–90.

STERLING, T. *ET AL.*, 'Typical pollutant concentrations in public buildings', in Perry, R. & Kirk, P. W. (eds.), *Indoor and Ambient Air Quality*, Proc. Indoor Amb. Air Quality Conf., Selper, London, 1988.
STERLING, T. *ET AL.*, 'ETS concentrations under different conditions of ventilation and smoking regulation', in *ibid.*

Biology and Common Sense

DE FRIES, J. F., 'Aging, natural death and the compression of morbidity', *New Engl. J. Med.*, 1980, 303(3): 130–5.
DU NOÜY, L., *Biological Time*, London, 1936.
RUDMAN, D., 'Nutrition and fitness in elderly people', *Am. J. Clin. Nutr.*, 1987, 49: 1090–8.

Philosophy of Life

SOCIALFORSKNINGSINSTITUTTETS *Social Sårbarhed og Modstandsdygtighed* (Social Vulnerability and Resistance). Publikation nr. 53, 1972.